OXFORD MEDICAL PUBLICATIONS

Pre-eclampsia

THE FACTS

D1344662

ALSO PUBLISHED BY OXFORD UNIVERSITY PRESS

Ageing: the facts (second edition)
Nicholas Coni, William Davidson, and Stephen Webster

Allergy: the facts
Robert J. Davies and Susan Oliver

Arthritis and rheumatism: the facts
J. T. Scott

Asthma: the facts (second edition)
Donald J. Lane and Anthony Storr

Back pain: the facts (second edition)
Malcolm Jayson

Bowel cancer: the facts
John M. A. Northover and Joel D. Kettner

Breast cancer: the facts (third edition)
Michael Baum (forthcoming)

Contraception: the facts (second edition)
Peter Bromwich and Tony Parsons

Coronary heart disease: the facts (second edition)
Desmond Julian and Claire Marley

Cystic fibrosis: the facts (second edition)
Ann Harris and Maurice Super

Deafness: the facts
Andrew P. Freeland

Down syndrome: the facts
Mark Selikowitz

Eating disorders: the facts (third edition)
S. Abraham and D. Llewellyn-Jones

Head injury: the facts
D. Gronwell, P. Wrightson, and P. Waddell

Kidney disease: the facts (second edition)
Stewart Cameron

Liver disease and gallstone: the facts (second edition)
A. G. Johnson and D. Triger

Lung cancer: the facts (second edition)
Chris Williams

Multiple sclerosis: the facts (second edition) Byran Matthews

Obsessive–compulsive disorder: the facts
Padmal de Silva and Sidney Rachman

Parkinson's disease: the facts (second edition)
Gerald Stern and Andrew Lees

Pre-eclampsia: the facts
Chris Redman and Isabel Walker

Thyroid disease: the facts (second edition)
R. I. S. Bayliss and W. M. G. Tunbridge

Pre-eclampsia

THE FACTS
The hidden threat to pregnancy

Chris Redman
Clinical Reader in Obstetric Medicine
John Radcliffe Hospital
Oxford

and

Isabel Walker
Medical journalist

Oxford   New York   Tokyo
OXFORD UNIVERSITY PRESS

Oxford University Press, Walton Street, Oxford OX2 6DP

Oxford New York Toronto
Delhi Bombay Calcutta Madras Karachi
Kuala Lumpur Singapore Hong Kong Tokyo
Nairobi Dar es Salaam Cape Town
Melbourne Auckland Madrid

and associated companies in
Berlin Ibadan

Oxford is a trade mark of Oxford University Press

Published in the United States
by Oxford University Press Inc., New York

First published 1992
Reprinted 1992

A catalogue record for this book is available from the British Library

Library of Congress Cataloging in Publication Data
Redman, Chris.
Pre-eclampsia: the facts: the hidden threat to pregnancy/
Chris Redman, Isabel Walker.
p. cm.—(Oxford medical publications)
1. Pre-eclampsia. I. Walker, Isabel. II. Title. III. Series.
(DNLM: 1. Pre-eclampsia–popular works. WQ 150 R318p)
RG575.5.R44 1992 618.7'5—dc20 91-31879

ISBN 0–19–262012–6 (h/b.)
ISBN 0–19–262013–4 (p/b.)

Printed in Great Britain by
Biddles Limited, Guildford and King's Lynn

To Benji and other 'lost' babies; and to all current and former patients of the Silver Star Unit in Oxford.

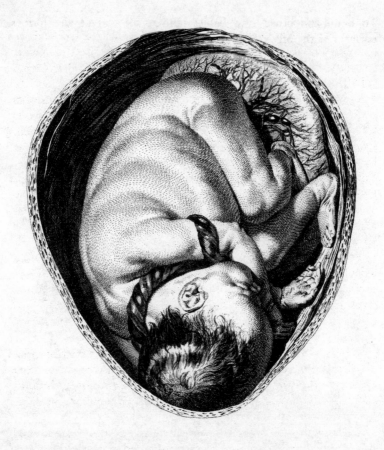

The unborn child (after William Smellie, the great 18th century Scottish obstetrician). The placenta—where pre-eclampsia originates—lies to one side of the baby, attached to the inner lining of the womb.

Preface

Pre-eclampsia is a clumsy, ugly word which means little or nothing to most women. Yet it is the most common and most dangerous complication of pregnancy, affecting more than 50 000 women a year in the UK alone.

One of us, a writer, has had a devastating personal experience of pre-eclampsia; the other, a doctor, has spent more than 20 years trying to make sense of this complex and mysterious condition. From our different perspectives we agreed that the little that *was* known about pre-eclampsia was clouded by ignorance, prejudice, and muddle. Doctors and midwives seemed confused by the very nature of the disease and pregnant women were cheerfully unaware of its existence—until a pre-eclamptic disaster struck. Then, always, the cry was the same: 'Why wasn't I warned? What did I do wrong? Why did this happen to me?'

When we looked for words of comfort and advice we found a complete dearth of information for public consumption. So we decided to write this book. We have pulled no punches and spared no details: we have assumed that the reader would be driven by a need to learn about the disease and would not be put off by technical detail and no-holds-barred descriptions of the worst cases.

We—and the book—have benefited enormously from the input of several hundred women who responded to a questionnaire on their experiences of pre-eclampsia. Many of their first-person accounts are scattered through the book to illustrate particular points more powerfully than mere description.

We hope that the book will prove useful not just to women—and their partners and families—who have suffered or might suffer pre-eclampsia, but also to midwives and general practitioners, who have the difficult task of screening for the disease in the community. If we can stimulate more awareness, understanding, and a greater sense of urgency about this problem, we will have achieved our aims.

Oxford C.R.
September 1991 I.W.

Acknowledgements

The authors wish to acknowledge the help of all the women who responded to the questionnaire which provided most of the case histories used in this book, and to thank the following publications which drew attention to the survey: *The Independent on Sunday*, *Living*, *She*, and *Mother*. We also wish to thank the following: Dr Irvine Loudon; Professor David Brock; Dr David Kilpatrick; Dr John Horvath; Dr Fiona Broughton Pipkin; Professor James Scott; Dr Iain Chalmers; Professor W. B. Robertson; Dawn James of The Pre-eclampsia Society (PETS); Andy Etchells for his unfailing professional advice and personal support; and all the obstetric and midwifery staff at the John Radcliffe Hospital, Oxford, who have, over many years, supported the development of a clinical and research interest in pre-eclampsia which has provided much of the material for this book.

Contents

1 · Introduction

Aileen Corner was only 27 weeks into her first pregnancy when suddenly, without warning, she suffered a convulsion which brought both her and her baby to the brink of disaster. She recalls:

I had enjoyed a perfectly normal pregnancy up until then. In fact, the day before I had been to an antenatal check and everything was OK. The next day I thought it was a bit strange when I couldn't fasten my maternity dress at the neck or get my shoes on, but I felt absolutely fine so I thought nothing more about it. That night when I went to bed a funny thing happened: every time I lay down I started to be sick, but when I sat up the feeling went away. It was so strange that we decided to call the doctor. He gave me a suppository to stop the sickness, after which I must have fallen asleep straightaway.

The next thing I knew my arms and legs were jerking and my husband literally dived out of bed with the shock. I shouted at him 'What's happening to me?'. Then I felt my head being flung back—and that's all I remember until 4 days later, when I woke up in the hospital intensive care unit to be shown a polaroid of a tiny baby in an incubator who they said was mine.

I had been taken to hospital by ambulance, where my blood pressure was found to be very high, and I was so ill that the baby had to be delivered urgently by Caesarean section. But the fits continued after delivery, and my heart was under such a strain that I had to spend a week in intensive care.

Paul weighed in at a healthy 4 lb 6 oz—my family has always produced big babies—but his weight quickly plummeted and he needed special care for 9 weeks. When they took me in a wheelchair to see him, the tears just ran down my face. He was so thin, covered with tubes and surrounded by monitors, all of them beeping, and I just couldn't believe this wee thing was mine. The doctors were surprised that he did so well considering he was so premature—but they said his size had a lot to do with it. He is now a healthy 6½-year-old.

As for me, I didn't understand what had happened, and even when the sister explained I wasn't much the wiser. Pre-eclampsia and eclampsia had never been mentioned in antenatal clinics, and I had seen no information about them in any books. I hadn't even heard the names before.

Most first-time mothers expect—and are led to expect—that if they are fit and well, with a good diet and a healthy lifestyle, they will sail through pregnancy with no problems at all. But for some, like Aileen, reality clashes so painfully with expectation that innocence and optimism are lost forever. Aileen suffered a rare and potentially lethal complication of pregnancy called *eclampsia*, which can strike at any time in the second half of pregnancy, during labour or in the first few days after delivery. The term describes convulsions and underlying disturbances, which are caused entirely by the pregnancy and only ever occur in women who are—or who very recently have been—pregnant.

Eclampsia is dangerous, frightening, and, fortunately, rare, affecting about 1 in every 2000 pregnant women in the UK. However, this adds up to more than 300 new cases every year, so Aileen's story, although dramatic and terrifying, is not unique.

Pre-eclampsia

What *is* unusual about Aileen's story is that her problems seemed to strike without warning. Most attacks of eclampsia are preceded by premonitory disturbances of growing severity. The cluster of disturbances are known collectively as *pre-eclampsia*.

Like eclampsia, pre-eclampsia is unique to pregnancy and can occur at any time from 20 weeks onwards. The condition, normally signalled by a combination of signs that may include raised blood pressure (*hypertension*), protein in the urine (*proteinuria*) and swelling (*oedema*), affects as many as 1 in 10 of all pregnancies if its milder forms are counted; it is particularly prevalent among first-time mothers, about 1 in 5 of whom is affected to some degree.

Most cases are mild, occurring at the very end of pregnancy and posing no threat to mother or child. But about 1 first-time mother in 20 suffers a more serious form of the disease, with reversible organ damage and blood clotting disturbances, as well as raised blood pressure. And about 1 in 100 first pregnancies is so severely affected that there is serious risk to the lives of the babies—and even their mothers!

So pre-eclampsia is common and dangerous—in fact, one of the most dangerous complications of human pregnancy. It is a leading cause of maternal death, killing around 10 women every year in the UK, and a major contributor to perinatal mortality, causing the deaths of up to 1000 babies every year. It is also the most important cause of prolonged antenatal hospitalization, of slow growth in otherwise normal singleton fetuses, and of induced premature delivery.

Pre-eclampsia is a world-wide problem, although it is impossible to compare national statistics because they are not routinely collected. Nevertheless, it is clear that developing countries with poor or non-existent antenatal care have higher death rates from pre-eclampsia and its complications than developed countries like the UK.

Given the prevalence and the risks of pre-eclampsia, one would have expected a high level of public awareness of the condition. Yet, paradoxically, it is a disease of which most mothers-to-be are almost entirely ignorant—until it strikes them.

When questioned in antenatal clinics, pregnant women are often remarkably well informed about such rare complications as Down syndrome and spina bifida, and the risks of German measles in pregnancy. But when asked about pre-eclampsia they tend to look blank, for the simple reason that *there is hardly any information available*. No leaflets are given out in antenatal clinics, although this one disease is the main justification for the endless checks on blood pressure, weight, and urine that form the cornerstone of antenatal care. Maternity handbooks offer reams of advice about backache, sickness, and constipation but appear curiously reluctant to burden their readers with this more serious concern. Parentcraft teachers tend to skip over the nine months of pregnancy in their rush to focus on the 'birth experience'.

Two factors underpin this low-profile treatment: first, pre-eclampsia is a complex, elusive, and unpredictable disease, which is so poorly understood by doctors themselves that they find it very difficult to offer much in the way of helpful information and advice. No-one understands the fundamental cause of the condition and so it is not possible, at present, to prevent or cure it—except by ending the pregnancy. Secondly, there is a tendency among some mothers-to-be to resist any bad news about pregnancy and to hear only what they want to hear. We live in the era of the 'designer pregnancy', when women are keen to tailor the experience to their own expectations, and modern catchphrases like 'pregnancy is not an illness' and 'childbirth should not be medicalized' tend to gloss over a very real health risk, which cannot be controlled by 'positive thinking' or any other consumerist approach.

It is not our intention to spread doom and gloom. Indeed, our overall message is positive: scientists are making great progress in unravelling the causes of pre-eclampsia; procedures are currently being tested that could lead to the prediction, prevention, and ultimately the eradication of the condition; the great majority of women who suffer severely in a first pregnancy are unaffected in subsequent pregnancies. However, it *is* our intention to redress the prevailing balance in favour of more information, coupled with more realistic expectations, so that mothers-to-be, armed with the necessary knowledge, can play the fullest possible part in helping to protect themselves against the worst consequences of this disease.

WHAT IS PRE-ECLAMPSIA?

Pre-eclampsia has been known by various names in the past, some of them still in use. The Victorians knew it as 'toxaemia of pregnancy', because they thought it was caused by one or more poisons circulating in the mother's bloodstream. This term is now obsolete, although a later description—'pre-eclamptic toxaemia'—persists, mostly because it can be conveniently abbreviated to PET.

'Pregnancy-induced hypertension' (PIH) is now a fashionable alternative to the term pre-eclampsia, although some doctors prefer 'hypertensive disease of pregnancy'. Both terms reflect the difficulty doctors experience in distinguishing pre-eclampsia from chronic hypertension that is revealed for the first time in pregnancy (see Chapter 4). Because of this, these terms are confusing and we do not use them in this book. Gestosis, a term meaning roughly the same as pre-eclampsia, is used widely in Europe but not in the UK.

Most diseases are defined by their causes. We know, for example, that heart disease is caused by progressive furring-up of the lining of the coronary arteries, while influenza is caused by a virus; but no-one knows what causes pre-eclampsia, so it is defined instead by the presence of a cluster of characteristic signs, none of which is unique to the disease on its own.

The signs of pre-eclampsia

The two major signs of pre-eclampsia are progressively rising blood pressure—a sign of circulatory disturbances—and the appearance of protein in the urine—a sign of kidney problems. Oedema—

generalized swelling caused by water retention—is a third, less reliable sign that is not always present and is, in any case, difficult to distinguish from the swelling associated with normal pregnancy.

The foundations for pre-eclampsia are thought to be laid in the first half of pregnancy, but the diagnostic signs do not normally appear until the final 3 months, which is why antenatal checks become more frequent at the start of the third trimester. However, in a minority of cases—and these are normally the most severe—the signs appear much earlier in the second half of pregnancy, when they risk going undetected because of the standard month-long intervals between antenatal check-ups at this stage of pregnancy.

Pre-eclampsia is believed to originate in the placenta, a shared organ, so it affects unborn babies as well as their mothers. The placenta's main task is to filter oxygen and nutrients from the mother's bloodstream to that of her baby; if the placenta is deficient, as it may be in pre-eclampsia, the baby's well-being and even its survival are threatened.

Characteristics

Pre-eclampsia has two key characteristics that make it very difficult to detect and manage. First it is a largely 'silent' disease, which in most cases causes no symptoms of illness at all. So it can only be reliably detected by 'screening' checks—regular, repetitive searches for the telltale signs in the final weeks of pregnancy. Secondly, pre-eclampsia always gets progressively worse as the pregnancy continues. Because nothing as yet can be done to halt or reverse this relentless progress, the only solution is to deliver the baby, which guarantees complete recovery to the mother in the vast majority of cases.

If a woman with severe pre-eclampsia does *not* have her baby delivered, she is at risk of such potentially lethal developments as eclampsia, cerebral haemorrhage, breakdown of the blood clotting system (disseminated intravascular coagulation) or liver failure, while her baby risks death in the womb from starvation or acute shortage of oxygen. The interests of mother and baby usually coincide, but sometimes it is necessary to save a mother at the expense of a baby who is too premature to survive delivery.

In theory, it should always be possible to protect mothers from the worst consequences of the disease by delivering their babies in good time. But in practice doctors can be caught out by the astonishing variability of pre-eclampsia. Some cases grumble on for months, while others appear to blow-up literally overnight, without warning. Some women have the classic signs while others don't appear to fit the bill. Some develop pre-eclampsia before they even *look* pregnant while others show the first signs during or just after delivery.

This difficulty in pinning pre-eclampsia down to a typical pattern is another reason why it is so hard to manage, and why it continues to be the major cause of the ultimate tragedy of pregnancy—maternal death.

WOMEN STILL DIE IN PREGNANCY

In the period 1952–4, the first years covered by the Government's triennial *Reports on Confidential Enquiries into Maternal Deaths in England and Wales*, 200 women died from pre-eclampsia or eclampsia, making them collectively the major cause of maternal death. In 1982–4, 25 women died of pre-eclampsia or eclampsia, and they were *still* the major cause of maternal death.

The deaths of 25 women in 3 years may not sound too drastic, and is nothing to the numbers who died of, say, cancer or heart disease in the same period. But these were healthy young women in the prime of their lives, setting out to create new life, not to lose their own. Death weighs heavily on the minds of people with diagnosed cancer or heart disease. But no-one expects to die in pregnancy—indeed the very idea is intolerable.

Of course, maternal death used to be quite common in the nineteenth and early twentieth centuries; but better health and nutrition, improved control of infection, and improved management of severe haemorrhage have made it a rarity. Even since 1952, maternal mortality in England and Wales has fallen more than 10-fold.

The pre-eclampsia-related deaths described in the *Confidential Enquiries* make uncomfortable reading, demonstrating as they do the lightning speed with which the disease can develop and progress to a disastrous conclusion in apparently healthy pregnant women. One woman mentioned in the 1982–4 report went into spontaneous labour at 32 weeks, showed the first signs of pre-eclampsia the next day, then collapsed within hours with a fatal cerebral haemorrhage. A second woman felt ill at 34 weeks, sent her husband to pick up a prescription from the GP, but died of cerebral haemorrhage before he returned. A third called her GP out because of vomiting and abdominal pain, and suffered repeated convulsions a few hours later, although the doctor had found nothing seriously wrong, then died within days.

More chilling than the descriptions of the deaths themselves is the clear implication that the majority were associated with substandard care by specialists.

'Care was considered substandard in 18 of the 25 deaths directly caused by hypertensive diseases of pregnancy,' states the report. But while the GP was thought culpable in five of these cases, the consultant team was judged to be at fault in all but two, either because they failed to diagnose the condition or because they failed to limit the damage and prevent major complications.

Most disturbing is the fact that, of the 14 women who died from eclampsia, seven had been admitted to a consultant unit *before* the first fit. Eclampsia is one of the most serious complications of severe pre-eclampsia, but it is nearly always preventable by good management, particularly a well-timed delivery. Yet these seven young women fell victim to fatal eclamptic fits under the care of 'experts'. There are no national statistics on the incidence of eclampsia and on what proportion of fits occur after admission to hospital. But undoubtedly many more similar cases occur without the tragic outcome.

What accounts for this substandard care, these failures of management? Undoubtedly it is a combination of the complexity of the condition and the comparative rarity of the most severe cases, which makes it difficult for specialists to gain enough experience to become skilled in managing the disease. The authors of the *Confidential Enquiries*, most of whom are eminent practising doctors, recognized as much when they called for the establishment of specialist regional teams, to which the most difficult cases could be referred (see Chapter 7).

THE GOOD NEWS

Clearly, there is a need for doctors, and particularly obstetricians, to provide better care for women with pre-eclampsia and eclampsia and to prevent all preventable tragedies. But the ultimate goal of everyone concerned with pre-eclampsia is to eradicate it completely by developing effective preventive measures.

The benefits of wiping out pre-eclampsia would be incalculable, not just to its potential victims but to all pregnant women and everyone working in the maternity services. Without the threat of pre-eclampsia, the number of antenatal visits required in the average pregnancy could be halved at a stroke; doctors and midwives would be free to devote their time and expertise to women who really need them; while the vast majority of mothers-to-be would be released to enjoy their pregnancies without interference.

The eradication of pre-eclampsia is a long-term prospect, which cannot happen until doctors and scientists have gained a better understanding of the disease they are trying to prevent. More is being learned about pre-eclampsia all the time: how the placenta becomes deficient, why this causes illness in the mother, and why the disease gets rapidly worse until the placenta is removed. But the answers to fundamental questions, like why the placental problem develops in the first place and what makes particular women prone to the disease and others not, are still not known.

Nevertheless, real and practical progress is being made on two important fronts:

Predictive testing

At present there is no reliable way of predicting who is and who is not at risk of pre-eclampsia, so the screening effort has to be diffused across the entire population of pregnant women. An accurate predictive test, which could be used early in pregnancy, would enable doctors to concentrate their efforts on clear 'high-risk' cases. Several possible tests are now being worked on (see Chapter 7, p. 151);

Prevention/delay

The most exciting recent development is the discovery that small daily doses of aspirin can delay, ameliorate, or even prevent pre-eclampsia in susceptible individuals. This theory has still to be substantiated by a large multinational trial, which is currently in progress, and doctors also need to be convinced that there is no risk of significant side-effects for pregnant women or their babies (see

Chapter 7). But if the news is good, it will be the biggest step forward for many many years.

It may be that by the end of the twentieth century, pre-eclampsia will have ceased to represent any real threat to pregnant women, so that they need know nothing about the disease. Unfortunately, at the moment it is too common, too dangerous, and too poorly understood for complacency, and *everybody* needs to know about it, which is why we have written this book.

2 · Pre-eclampsia in perspective

The north wall of the chancel of Buxton Church in Norfolk houses a memorial tablet with the following inscription, couched in the florid Latin phraseology of the age of Charles I:

Here lies Margaret Robinson, daughter of Arthur Robinson, Knight, of the county of York, and wife of Robert Jegon Esquire with whom she was joined in the most chaste bond of married love for the space of nine years and, after she had most happily given birth to five children, her sixth offspring died while still enclosed in her womb. After being shaken by the force of frequent convulsions, she gave up her soul to heaven on the fourth day of December AD 1638.

This is a clear case of eclampsia, and one of the earliest on record. Of course, the poor woman had probably been suffering from pre-eclampsia for some time before the onset of these fatal fits, but neither she nor her advisers would have had any way of knowing this: there were no blood pressure machines, no dipstick urine tests, indeed no antenatal checks at all in the seventeenth century, and even if Margaret Robinson's illness *had* been recognized for what it was, there would have been no safe way of delivering her baby early to arrest its fatal course.

In fact, the disease we now know as pre-eclampsia was not identified until two centuries after Margaret Robinson's tragic demise, and it was to be another hundred years before babies could be safely induced or delivered by Caesarean section to save their own or their mothers' lives.

The susceptibility of pregnant women to convulsions was known to ancient civilizations, but it was not until the eighteenth century that eclampsia, which is specific to pregnancy, was distinguished from epilepsy, a chronic recurring condition, which can affect anyone at any time of life.

For some time after this, eclampsia was assumed to be a sudden event arising without warning. Only in the midnineteenth century, when premonitory signs began to be identified, was a 'pre-eclamptic' syndrome recognized, although it was not given that name. It was not until the middle of the twentieth century that pre-eclampsia was well enough defined to be separated from the unrelated chronic illnesses that it resembles, although even now confusion persists over the distinction between some forms of chronic hypertension, detected for the first time in pregnancy, and the pregnancy-induced high blood pressure of pre-eclampsia.

Theories about what causes the condition have ranged from bacterial infection to epilepsy, from external irritants to internal toxins, from overeating to malnutrition, from liver disease to kidney disease, and from repletion (too much blood flowing to the brain) to depletion (its opposite). Treatments over the centuries have been correspondingly diverse, including bleeding and purging, starvation, sedation, paralysis, diuresis, sweating, dietary manipulation, drainage of the spinal fluid, removal of the ovaries, and even mastectomy!

DEFINING THE DISEASE

References to fits in pregnancy or around delivery are alleged to appear in ancient Egyptian, Chinese, and Indian writings, but the first convincing allusion, according to biochemist Leon C. Chesley, the US authority on pre-eclampsia, is to be found in the pre-Hippocratic *Coan Prognosis* of the ancient Greeks. This stated, in a way that comes near to anticipating pre-eclampsia: 'In pregnancy, the onset of drowsy headaches with heaviness is bad; such cases are perhaps liable to some sort of fits at the same time.'

Hippocrates in the fourth century BC, Celsus, a Roman, in the first century AD, Galen, a Greek physician in Rome in the second century AD, and Aetios of Almida, a Greek physician in the sixth century AD, all referred to life-threatening convulsions in pregnancy. Much later, in the sixteenth century, the German physician Gaebelkhouern identified four different types of epilepsy, one of which originated in the pregnant uterus, particularly if occupied by a malformed fetus. Mothers in these circumstances, he said, feel a biting and gnawing in the uterus and diaphragm—a description that some modern commentators have taken as a reference to the epigastric (upper abdominal) pain, which is a classic symptom of very severe pre-eclampsia.

It might seem strange that such a spectacular and terrifying event as an eclamptic fit should attract so few references over the centuries but there are two very good explanations for this. First, eclampsia had not yet been distinguished from epilepsy, and so was not remarkable in itself; secondly, the distinguished doctors responsible for chronicling their times were male, and obstetrics was almost exclusively in the hand of female midwives. The modern literature of eclampsia began in France in the late seventeenth century, when male obstetricians first made their mark.

The most eminent of this new breed was François Mauriceau, who made the following entry in his *Observations Grossesse*:

On 23 March 1669 I was called to deliver a woman of twenty-five, in labour with her first child. She had been taken with furious convulsions for a day and a half, losing all consciousness and had almost bitten off her tongue with her teeth.

Mauriceau did not explicitly differentiate these 'furious convulsions' from epilepsy, but he obviously recognized them as being specific to pregnancy because he attributed them either to an excess of heated blood from the uterus or to malignant vapours arising from the decomposition of a dead fetus. Mauriceau set out several 'aphorisms' on the subject, which have since been proved substantially true: first-time mothers are most at risk; convulsions during pregnancy are more dangerous than those beginning after delivery; fits are most dangerous when the fetus is already dead; the danger to both mother and baby is greatest when the mother does not recover consciousness between convulsions.

Eclampsia was first distinguished from epilepsy in 1739 by another Frenchman, Bossier de Sauvages, who reserved the 'epilepsy' label for chronic, recurring convulsions and introduced 'eclampsia' to describe all convulsions with a one-off causation, including pain, haemorrhage and parasitic infestation as well as pregnancy/childbirth.

The origins of the word 'eclampsia' are controversial. Some authorities say it is derived from a Greek word meaning something like 'a flash of lightning' or 'a bolt from the blue' but others argue that it is simply a translation for epilepsy. Whatever its derivation, the word itself has stuck, although it was not until the midtwentieth century that the definition was restricted to convulsions in pregnancy/childbirth and the immediate postnatal period.

The first hint that signs other than convulsions were associated with eclampsia came in 1797, when the French obstetrician

Demanet drew attention to oedema in a series of six eclamptic patients and argued that this was a cause of their convulsions.

A greater step forward occurred in Britain, in 1843, when Dr John Lever showed that eclampsia was associated with large amounts of protein in the urine. Lever found proteinuria in nine out of a series of ten convulsive women—and a later postmortem on the tenth showed she had acute meningitis, not eclampsia. By this time, according to Oxford medical historian Dr Irvine Loudon, other signs, including oedema, blurred vision, and headaches were recognized as precursors of eclampsia, and Lever was able to show that women with these warning signs were also proteinuric.

Lever's discovery at first suggested that the fits were related to nephritis (kidney inflammation), which was also characterized by oedema and proteinuria. Indeed the delusion that pre-eclampsia/eclampsia was a form of kidney disease prevailed for most of the next hundred years—and even persists to this day among some specialists.

Hypertension, the sign that most doctors think of as a *sine qua non* for a diagnosis of pre-eclampsia, was not recognized until the turn of the twentieth century, when it became possible to measure arterial pressure indirectly by means of sphygmomanometry—the method still in current use. It soon became clear that the blood pressure was significantly raised not only in eclamptic women but also in those who had not convulsed but who had proteinuria. Thus the concept of pre-eclampsia was born, although the issue was still blurred by the confusion with kidney disease, which can also cause high blood pressure.

In recent years, much more knowledge has been amassed about the different signs of the disease and the various forms of damage it can wreak. For example, doctors now know that pre-eclampsia does not affect just the circulatory system (hypertension) or indeed the kidneys (proteinuria), but can disturb the clotting system, the liver, the brain, the vision, the lungs, the heart, and potentially every organ and system in the body.

At the same time, precise ultrasound techniques have demonstrated how the unborn baby is affected by pre-eclampsia, giving rise to the modern idea that the disease is shared by mother and baby, although their symptoms are completely different.

A DISEASE OF THEORIES

In the 250-odd years since eclampsia was named, dozens of theories have been put forward to explain the origin of the disease but not a single one has been proved. 'As a matter of fact,' said the American Joseph B. De Lee in 1904—and he might as well have said it yesterday:

we know practically nothing of the causation of eclampsia. A theory has only to be set up by one investigator to be knocked down by another, and since there are a large number of theories advanced, we must give both sets of workers credit for the immense amount of labor and time consumed in building up these theories and in knocking them down.

Before eclampsia was recognized as an entity in its own right, doctors accepted the Hippocratic view that convulsions were caused in some circumstances by repletion (too much blood flowing to the brain) and in others by the opposite, depletion. It was the discovery of proteinuria in eclamptic patients in the midnineteenth century, and the apparent link with kidney disease, which sparked off the great proliferation of theories about the possible origins of the condition.

Most of these theories are not worth examining here: they include compression of the ureters (the tubes carrying urine from the kidneys to the bladder); hypersensitivity of the nervous system to external irritants; bacterial infection; inflammation of the womb lining; irritation of the uterus, and thyroid malfunction. However, two theories that gained particular credence in their time, and which are worth outlining at length, are the kidney diseases theory and the 'toxaemia' theory.

The kidney disease theory

The concept of eclampsia as a kidney disease was first developed in the midnineteenth century after Lever discovered proteinuria in his eclamptic patients. Lever himself concluded that eclampsia was different from nephritis because the proteinuria abated rapidly after delivery. But his contemporaries were confused by the fact that one woman who died of eclampsia *did* have chronic nephritis, and was therefore found to have damaged kidneys at postmortem.

In 1851, the German physician Frerichs published an influential book, in which he argued that eclampsia was a form of uraemia—

the end stage of nephritis. In uraemia, excessive amounts of urea and other waste products normally excreted by the kidneys accumulate in the blood with toxic effects. This theory gained credence despite the fact that postmortems carried out on women who had died of eclampsia often uncovered no apparent renal abnormalities.

Towards the end of the nineteenth century, a form of liver damage that is characteristic of pre-eclampsia/eclampsia was detected for the first time, so allowing the condition to be distinguished from nephritis. Nevertheless, the confusion with kidney disease persisted until well into the twentieth century.

It is now known that although women with pre-existing kidney disease are particularly prone to pre-eclampsia, pre-eclampsia itself is not primarily a kidney disease. The proteinuria that marks the onset of severe disease is one of pre-eclampsia's many *effects*, not its causes.

The toxaemia theory

The toxaemia theory—that pre-eclampsia/eclampsia is caused by one or more poisons circulating in the mother's bloodstream—also surfaced in the midnineteenth century. The earliest reference known to Chesley (see p. 11) is by William Tyler Smith, who wrote in 1849:

It deserves to be borne in mind that the depurgatory functions ought, in order to preserve health, to be increased during gestation, as the debris of the foetal as well as the maternal system have to be eliminated by the organs of the mother. Besides *these forms of toxaemia* [our italics], the state of the blood which obtains during fevers, or during the excitement of the first secretion of milk, may excite the convulsive disorder.

The dawn of the twentieth century witnessed almost unanimous agreement that 'the convulsive disorder' was caused by a circulating toxin. In his 1904 round-up of past and current theories, Dr Lee concluded:

. . . only one point seems to be generally conceded, namely that eclampsia is due to the action of a toxin in the blood upon the nerve centers. How and where the toxin is formed are unknown.

The various potential toxins put forward at one time or another have included water; fetal waste products; bacterial toxins; toxins released by the placenta, or even by the fetus itself; substances normally excreted in menstruation and therefore retained during pregnancy; and normal waste products retained in the body because of impaired function of various excretory organs.

At first it was thought that a whole range of pregnancy complications could be caused by one or more toxins; thus the term 'toxaemias of pregnancy' referred not just to pre-eclampsia but also to excessive vomiting (*hyperemesis*), gingivitis, herpes, placental abruption, and hypertension from any cause. At the turn of the twentieth century, pre-eclampsia was commonly referred to as 'the' toxaemia of pregnancy.

Some experts believed that a single toxin was responsible for all the various toxaemias, others that a different toxin was responsible for each separate disorder. Either way, the word 'toxaemia', was used in official classifications until the 1950s and indeed many doctors still use the term 'pre-eclamptic toxaemia' or PET.

Although no toxin that could conceivably be responsible for pre-eclampsia has even been identified, the toxaemia theory is not completely dead and may even be due for a revival. Many experts now believe that the maternal illness in pre-eclampsia is directly caused by a substance—known, until it is identified, as 'factor X'—which is released into the mother's bloodstream by a deficient placenta.

The importance of the placenta in the evolution of pre-eclampsia was recognized many years ago. As early as 1914 the Edinburgh physician Dr James Young produced: '. . . evidence to support the view that the eclamptic phenomenon has as its immediate cause a massive damage of the placenta'. Unfortunately, damage of the sort he described was not always evident in placentas examined after delivery, so his theories were disregarded. They were revived in 1948 by the American obstetrician Ernest Page, who argued that the placenta did not have to be grossly damaged to cause pre-eclampsia—just kept short of maternal blood; and this remains the theory most widely accepted today.

TREATMENT

The treatment of pre-eclampsia through the ages has been as fascinatingly eclectic as the underlying theories of causation, but the very length of the list of medical procedures that have been used singly or in combination since the early nineteenth century suggests what doctors now know to be true—nothing actually *works* except delivery.

As the American obstetricians Zuspan and Ward wrote in 1964, the pre-eclamptic patient has over the centuries been:

. . . blistered, bled, purged, packed, lavaged, irrigated, punctured, starved, sedated, anaesthetised, paralysed, tranquillized, rendered hypotensive, drowned, been given diuretics, had mammectomy, been dehydrated, forcibly delivered and neglected.

Chesley has since added to this list of insults with a range of surgical procedures, including implantation of the ureters in the colon, renal decapsulation (stripping of the membrane that envelops the kidney), drainage of spinal fluid, ventral suspension of the uterus, (stitching it to the abdominal wall), postpartum curettage (scraping away the womb lining), and removal of the ovaries.

The mainstays of treatment of eclampsia until the midnineteenth century were bleeding and purging. Bleeding seemed a logical treatment when eclampsia was thought to be caused by excessive blood flow to the brain. Later, when the toxaemia theory gained credence, bleeding still appeared appropriate because, in theory, it helped to rid the body of whatever was poisoning it. It also made sense in this context to stimulate the body's other excretory functions, so the use of diuretic, purgative, emetic, and sweat-inducing drugs also became popular after the midnineteenth century, along with procedures to 'wash-out' the stomach and intestines.

Later in the nineteenth century, heavy sedation with narcotic and anaesthetic drugs was added to the earlier measures; and some doctors used a primitive and risky form of induction known as forced delivery, which involved rupturing the membranes and then inserting a device into the lower part of the uterus to stimulate contractions.

Towards the end of the nineteenth century treatment began to polarize between two extremes: doctors in Holland and Germany advocated active obstetric interference in the form of Caesarean section, which gradually replaced induction for severe cases; while doctors in Dublin and Russia adopted ultraconservative medical regimes, keeping their patients heavily sedated and waiting for labour to begin spontaneously.

Caesarean section was the more popular treatment in the USA, as well as in Germany and Holland, but the results in the early twentieth century were not good—the operation was not nearly as safe as it is now and eclamptic women were often not admitted to hospital for many hours, even days, after the onset of convulsions, by which time they were too ill to survive the operation.

In 1922 the eminent London obstetrician Thomas Watts Eden compared the results of Caesarean delivery with those of natural delivery, assisted delivery, and induction and found little for the advocates of intervention to congratulate themselves about. While the death rate for mothers who had a natural delivery was 4.5 per cent for 'mild' eclampsia and 36.9 for severe disease, the figures rose to 11.3 per cent and 46.3 per cent, respectively, for mothers delivered by Caesarean section. 'These results constitute a very powerful plea for restraint in the obstetric management of cases of eclampsia,' he said. 'Active interference as represented by Caesarean section . . . diminishes the patient's chances of recovery instead of increasing them.'

The keystone of the alternative conservative management regimes was sedation. In Dublin, Tweedy kept his patients sedated and starved while bleeding, purging, and washing-out to remove toxins. When labour started, forceps were applied as soon as they could be pushed through the cervix.

Meanwhile, Stroganoff, in Russia, rendered his patients almost comatose with sedative drugs and kept them under constant observation in quiet, darkened rooms. This treatment continued up to and including labour and for 24 hours after delivery. When the cervix was 6 cm dilated, the membranes were ruptured artificially and delivery was often assisted with forceps.

Tweedy, and especially Stroganoff, reported marked reductions in maternal mortality in comparison with more radical methods, and gradually won converts. The pendulum swung more heavily in their direction after the disappointing results of Caesarean section became known; and for a while obstetric intervention went completely out of favour, as seriously ill eclamptic women were allowed to continue with pregnancies for weeks after the onset of convulsions, leading to a soaring rate of stillbirths. Eventually, a better balance was struck between conservative treatment and intervention, but these situations remained fraught with danger until the advent of safe induction and Caesarean section in the latter half of the twentieth century.

Meanwhile, the Americans had discovered another form of conservative treatment involving the injection of magnesium sulphate, the main constituent of Epsom's salts and a well-known laxative when taken orally. Its use in the prevention of eclampsia at first seemed bizarre, yet it is now the routine treatment for eclampsia in the US and other parts of the Western hemisphere, with the noteable exception of the UK. The treatment has never really taken off in the UK, partly through historical accident, but also because it has never been clear *how* the drug works in preventing eclampsia.

The injection of magnesium sulphate to control the convulsions of eclampsia was first reported in 1904 by a Norwegian doctor who delivered the drug directly into the fluid around the spinal cord. But it was an American obstetrician Lazard who pioneered its infusion through a vein, and this has become the mainstay of treatment in the US. In 1925 he wrote: 'Our experience in the few cases here reported has been so uniformly successful that we feel that it is worthy of further and more extensive trial . . .' Such a trial was soon carried out by the US obstetrician McNeile, who reported a three-fold reduction in maternal mortality associated with eclampsia, from 36.2 to 12 per cent.

Drugs to reduce high blood pressure—known as *antihypertensives* —were introduced in the 1950s. The first to be used widely was hydralazine, which proved rapidly effective when given by injection, and was incorporated into routine practice as the potentially lethal effects of uncontrolled hypertension became clear. Other antihypertensive drugs were introduced subsequently as soon as their safety in pregnancy could be demonstrated, but they were not widely used in the management of pre-eclampsia until the 1970s, when it was shown that they could help to prolong affected pregnancies.

Diuretics were fashionable in the 1960s, and were prescribed to prevent and treat the swelling caused by fluid retention. They seemed to be just what was needed: safe, potent, and almost magical in their ability to restore an oedematous woman's shape to near normal. However, they offered no solution to the underlying problem, and eventually the pendulum of fashion swung away to the point that they were considered almost dangerous (see Chapter 5).

Control of fluid retention by salt restriction was also popular in the 1950s, but in 1958 this was shown to be dangerous, and has since fallen into disrepute.

Probably the greatest advance of the twentieth century has been the development of safe, effective methods of induction. This was facilitated in the 1960s and 1970s by the introduction of uterine-stimulating drugs and the advent of safe Caesarean sections as a back-up. These days, early delivery poses minimal risks to the mother, while babies are at risk only on account of their prematurity.

PROGRESS TOWARDS PREVENTION

It was not until well into the twentieth century that any progress was made in reducing the unacceptably high toll of maternal deaths from pre-eclampsia/eclampsia.

The figures speak eloquently for themselves: In England and Wales between 1872 and 1876 there were just over 5400 maternal deaths for every million births, of which 630 were caused by 'toxaemia'. In 1933, when total maternal mortality had fallen slightly to 4510 per million births, 760 were attributed to toxaemia. It would probably be unfair to interpret this as a rise in toxaemia-related deaths, as it is certain that more cases of pre-eclampsia were being recognized in 1933. Nevertheless, there was clearly no significant *improvement*, despite such advances as Caesarean section, improved teaching of obstetrics and growing provision of antenatal care.

The mainstays of so-called preventive treatment in the nineteenth century were bleeding and special diets—particularly those low in meat protein. As early as 1824 the French physician Miquel was recommending a bland milky diet to stave off maternal convulsions. In the latter half of the century low-protein diets were advocated for an ever-increasing number of reasons: they were thought to minimize gastric irritation, which might help to trigger convulsions; they reduced the burden of excretion for the kidneys; they were low in so-called 'toxins'.

A marked decrease in the incidence of eclampsia in Germany during the First World War, coinciding with a shortage of meat, appeared to bolster the case for low-protein diets. In 1917 an editorial in the authoritative *Journal of the American Medical Association* commented: 'The conclusion seems inevitable that restrictions of fat and meat tend to ward off eclampsia'.

The low-protein diet theory was taken seriously for a long time and was still being advocated as late as 1945. However, there has never been any reliable evidence for the efficacy of such a diet and nutritionists are now much more likely to urge a higher-than-normal intake of protein in pregnancy.

The most significant measure for preventing the worst consequences of pre-eclampsia has been the widespread introduction of antenatal care, geared to detecting the warning signs of the condition at an early stage and pre-empting its progression by early delivery.

Antenatal care for all was introduced gradually after the First World War, with the prime aim of reducing maternal mortality from all causes, which had remained steady since the midnineteenth century despite a consistent fall in the overall death rate. The need to screen for pre-eclampsia dictated the content and pattern of the checks, which have been maintained for the last 60 years.

The first hospital out-patient antenatal clinic in Britain opened in 1915 at Edinburgh's Royal Maternity Hospital. By 1935 it was estimated that 80 per cent of all expectant mothers received antenatal care of some kind, nearly half of them in state-aided clinics. However, the 1930s were a time of disillusionment, when it became clear that the widespread provision of antenatal care had done nothing to reduce maternal mortality. In 1934 a leading article in *The Lancet* declared:

A serious criticism of antenatal care is to be found in our failure to reduce the death rate from toxaemia . . . Considering that eclampsia is almost entirely a preventable disease, the incidence and death rate are still far too high.

According to Sir Alec Turnbull in *Obstetrics* (Churchill Livingstone, 1989) the persistently high maternal mortality was most probably due to poor obstetric care, including an astonishingly high prevalence of forceps deliveries carried out by poorly trained GPs under chloroform or other forms of anaesthesia.

Only when antenatal provision was matched by a high standard of obstetric care could mothers reap its rewards. The great twentieth century decline in maternal mortality may have been sparked off by the widespread introduction of sulphonamides (early antibiotics) but was most probably sustained by better care. 'In England and Wales, maternal mortality finally began to fall around 1937,' says Turnbull:

. . . and when it did, the fall was sudden, profound, and sustained, continuing up to the present time. There have been few more remarkable statistical changes during the twentieth century. The same fall occurred in all the developed countries, in Europe, Scandinavia and the USA at the same time.

The rate of improvement in maternal mortality has been constant, approximately halving every 10 years. From over 4000 deaths per million births in 1937, the rate had fallen to 86 per million by 1982–4.

Changes in the death rate from pre-eclampsia/eclampsia are less thoroughly documented, partly because of problems of definition. But it *is* known that in England and Wales in 1920, 780 deaths per million confinements were ascribed to 'puerperal convulsions' (eclampsia) or 'albuminuria of pregnancy' (pre-eclampsia). In the period 1952–4 the maternal mortality rate for pre-eclampsia/ eclampsia was just under 120 per million maternities, falling more or less steadily to the current level of just over 13 per million.

There is no suggestion that the incidence of pre-eclampsia has fallen since the 1930s; but eclampsia, which is in most cases a preventable complication of pre-eclampsia, is nowhere near as common as it used to be. There are no national statistics, but local reports produced in the UK and overseas document a marked downward trend.

For example, a study carried out in Aberdeen showed that cases of eclampsia among first-time mothers fell from 0.8 per cent in 1938–42 to 0.3 per cent in 1951–3. A report from New Zealand, where eclampsia was a notifiable disease, showed a fall in incidence from 3.2 per 1000 total births in 1928–33 to 1.39 in 1940–6 and to 0.80 in 1956–8; over the same period, the associated mortality rate fell more than five-fold, from 18.9 to 3.5 per cent.

The fall in the perinatal mortality rate (stillbirths and deaths in the first week after birth) began later. Perinatal mortality has been falling consistently since the late 1950s in England and Wales, from 35 deaths per 1000 births in 1958 to fewer than 9 per 1000 in 1987.

It is difficult to chart national shifts in perinatal mortality associated with pre-eclampsia as these deaths are often attributed to other causes, noteably prematurity. But a revealing picture was given by a local study, published in 1977, which charted changes in the perinatal death rate from pre-eclampsia in Aberdeen between 1948 and 1973. Despite a very high standard of antenatal care from 1948 onwards, there was no fall in the perinatal mortality rate from pre-eclampsia in first births between 1948 and 1964. Indeed, the rate rose from around 5 per 1000 births in 1948 to a sharp peak of 7.5 per 1000 in 1963. However, the rate declined rapidly after 1964, reaching 2 per 1000 by 1967 and remaining just above that level thereafter. This dramatic fall coincided with such advances as a greater ability to assess the well-being of babies in the womb, an increased understanding of how the baby is involved in the pre-eclamptic process and a growing willingness to terminate affected pregnancies in the baby's interests, coupled with the advent of safer Caesarean sections and more effective induction techniques.

Much of the modern management of pre-eclampsia dates from an influential report by Australian obstetrician, John Hamlin, working in Sydney. In *The Lancet* in 1952 he made the startling claim that he had 'eliminated' eclampsia in his hospital by introducing a system of rigidly enforced antenatal supervision.

This involved putting all his patients on high-protein diets, admitting them to hospital as soon as they showed the earliest signs of pre-eclampsia and then delivering them before complications could develop. Noting how the worst disasters appeared to befall those who defaulted on their clinic visits, he resorted to drastic measures to force them to attend:

'The nearest police station was telephoned and the police were asked to deliver the message that an immediate visit to the hospital was expected. Excellent results followed this procedure in most instances.'

Hamlin's paper illuminated the three key principles by which pre-eclampsia is still controlled today: early diagnosis, early admission to hospital, and well-timed delivery.

Pre-eclampsia now

Contradictory opinions about the definition, causes, treatment, and prevention of pre-eclampsia have been a constant feature of the history of the disease. The controversies stemmed, of course, from ignorance. Unless ideas are anchored to firm, irrefutable facts they can be distorted by opinions, prejudices, fears, and imagination.

Later in this book we will describe how new and reliable information is illuminating and clarifying modern perceptions of pre-eclampsia. But first we need to go back to basics: what happens in normal pregnancy—and how does it all go wrong in pre-eclampsia?

3 · Portrait of a normal pregnancy

Pre-eclampsia is a complex, multifaceted and enormously variable condition, which is not fully understood, even by acknowledged experts. However, most authorities agree that it arises as a result of partial failure of the unique 'partnership' between a pregnant woman and her unborn child.

We can only begin to appreciate the implications of this failure by first understanding how this partnership is *supposed* to operate and *does* work in a normal pregnancy; that is what this chapter is about.

Most of us have only a hazy idea of how the mother's body supports and nurtures the growing baby. We may be aware that the placenta plays a crucial role in transporting oxygen and nutrients from the mother's bloodstream to that of her baby, but we are largely ignorant of the profound and dramatic changes in maternal physiology, which enable this finely balanced interchange to take place.

To meet the needs of the developing pregnancy, extra blood has to be pumped around the body and the blood vessels—particularly those supplying the placenta—must expand to carry it; the blood composition changes so that it can clot more easily in case of haemorrhage; the heart works harder, as do the kidneys and lungs, which must excrete extra waste chemicals and gases from the baby; the mother has to lay down extra fat, absorb more nutrients from her food, and mobilize her nutritional stores to meet her baby's needs.

These and many other changes are all part of the normal maternal adaptation to pregnancy and it is part of the miracle of reproduction that they happen not in *reaction* to the growing baby's demands but in *anticipation*. Most of these changes are set in motion at the very earliest stage of pregnancy, around the time of implantation of the fertilized egg into the uterine wall.

THE MYSTERY OF IMPLANTATION

The female egg is fertilized in the outer end of the fallopian tube, near the ovary. After fertilization it travels slowly along the tube, to enter the uterus 3 or 4 days later. In the course of this journey, first the fertilized egg divides into two smaller cells then, about 15 hours after this first division, both cells divide in two, to give four even smaller cells, and so on, until by the time the cell cluster enters the uterus it comprises about 64 cells.

This cell cluster is no bigger than the original egg and is still contained within the egg's original coating, the *zona pellucida*. Only a few of these early cells will go on to form the baby; most will develop into the placenta and its membranes.

Shortly after entering the uterus, the cluster reshapes itself into a hollow, fluid-filled ball of cells, which 'hatches' as an embryo from the zona pellucida and is ready to attach itself to the innermost lining of the uterus, known in pregnancy as the *decidua*.

Implantation begins about a week after fertilization, when the outermost layer of embryonic cells, known as the *trophoblast*, first anchors the embryo to the decidua and then begins to burrow into the maternal tissue, feeding the embryo on the rich mixture of blood and secretions within.

The precise mechanisms controlling implantation are not well understood, although it is known that the hormones progesterone (secreted by the mother's ovaries after ovulation) and chorionic gonadotrophin (secreted by the embryo itself) both help to make the womb lining thick, nourishing, and receptive.

THE IMMUNE SYSTEM

The partnership that begins with implantation is remarkable and paradoxical: for the next 9 months the baby will grow attached to and supported by the tissues of its mother's womb; yet these tissues, especially in the first trimester, are packed with immune cells, whose normal function is to protect the body from invasion by alien organisms.

An efficient immune system is essential for good health, tracking down and destroying the great majority of infective organisms without the help of drugs. This policing function is made possible by the immune system's unique ability to spot the difference between cells which do and do not belong in the body. So precise and comprehensive is this discriminatory capacity that it cannot tolerate the presence in the body of cells from any other individual except a genetically identical twin. This is why transplanted organs are so prone to 'rejection'.

The newly implanted embryo, known to scientists as 'nature's transplant', is foreign on account of its paternal genes, and should by rights be rejected. Yet this does not happen—despite the fact that the mother's immune system remains in otherwise perfect working order throughout pregnancy.

Immunologists have recognized and been puzzled by this central paradox of pregnancy for more than 35 years. By what means does a mother's immune system continue to do its normal work yet tolerate the presence of the growing baby? Might there be circumstances in which problems, such as pre-eclampsia, arise because of a breakdown in this balancing act?

THE PLACENTAL 'TREE' AND THE TWO CIRCULATIONS

Even before implantation, the cells of the early embryo have separated into two types: the inner cell mass, which will become the baby and its protective membranes, and the outer cells, which are known collectively as the trophoblast.

The trophoblast

The trophoblast, the only embryonic tissue that comes into direct contact with maternal tissue, has several functions: its main purpose is to form the placenta, the plate-shaped organ that juxtaposes the maternal and fetal circulations so that oxygen and nutrients can pass from mother to baby and waste products from baby to mother. The placenta does not become fully established until the end of the first trimester of pregnancy.

A secondary function of the trophoblast, and one that is crucial to the success of the pregnancy, is to engineer structural changes in the tiny maternal blood vessels terminating in the placental bed— the part of the uterus to which the placenta is attached—so that they can carry an ever-increasing volume of blood to the placenta. These vessels are known as 'spiral arteries', because of their coiled shape, and there are about 150 of them supplying the placenta. The trophoblast cells remodel these arteries to meet the needs of the pregnancy by breaking down their musculo-elastic walls and turning them into passive, funnel-shaped vessels with a hugely increased capacity.

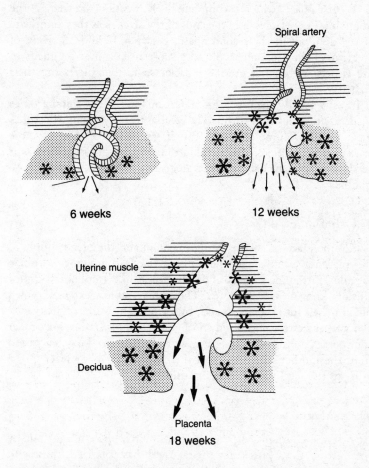

Fig. 3.1   A diagram of how invading placental cells create the placenta's blood supply from the small spiral arteries of the uterus. The cells (black stars) infiltrate the arteries' walls and cause them to thin out, allowing the vessels to enlarge and conduct much more blood. In pre-eclampsia the process of enlargement of blood vessels never seems to progress beyond the stage reached at 12 weeks. This means that the arteries end up too small to transmit enough blood to the placenta, which then becomes ischaemic at some point in the second half of pregnancy.

The spiral arteries (Fig. 3.1)

The transformation of the spiral arteries takes place in two phases: in the first phase, which is complete by 12 weeks of pregnancy, the trophoblast penetrates only the ends of the arteries as they terminate in the decidua; in the second phase, between 12 and 18 weeks of pregnancy, the trophoblast invades more deeply into segments of the vessels within the uterine muscle, so further increasing their capacity.

If, as is usually the case, this transformation of the spiral arteries is successful, they will ultimately be able to carry about 100 times their normal volume of blood. But if, as sometimes happens, the process is incomplete, the placenta cannot get as much blood as it needs to supply the baby and the pregnancy will eventually run into trouble.

The chorionic villi

While the placental bed is being prepared and the blood supply to the placenta established, the embryo itself is growing within a capsule, surrounded on all sides by frond-like trophoblastic protrusions known as *chorionic villi*. The embryo rapidly extends its own blood vessels into these villi and, by about eight weeks of pregnancy —six weeks after conception and five after implantation—a proper transport system has been set up, with nutrients and oxygen passed from the mother's blood, across the outer trophoblast layer of the villi, to the fetal blood vessels within.

The placenta

At first the chorionic villi completely encircle the embryo, but by the 12th week of pregnancy their growth has polarized; those villi growing into the uterus at the site of the original implantation become the placenta, while the rest gradually shrivel and are incorporated into the membranes encircling the baby. After the 14th week the placenta is fully established and ready to take over the function of nourishing the baby via the blood vessels of the umbilical cord.

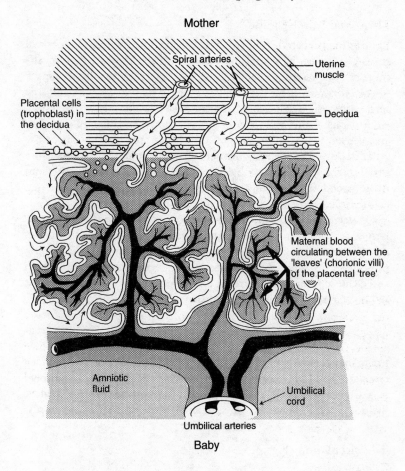

Fig. 3.2 The placenta 'tree'. Diagram (not to scale) of the branching structure of the placenta. For simplicity, the veins that always accompany the arteries are not shown.

For the rest of the pregnancy, the placenta grows with the baby. To imagine what it looks like, it is helpful to think of a tree: the umbilical cord attaching the baby to the placenta is the trunk; this gives way to many close-packed branching vessels at the tips of which are densely interwoven 'leaves' in the form of the chorionic villi.

The placental 'tree' (Fig. 3.2)

Each villus is coated with trophoblast and filled with a network of small capillaries, which receive blood from the baby via the umbilical cord. Between the branches and leaves of the placenta is a space —the *intervillous space*—which is bathed in maternal blood from the spiral arteries. Here, a fine balancing act is achieved, with the two circulations—mother's and baby's—brought intimately together and yet kept totally separate by the thin trophoblastic coat of the villi. Dissolved oxygen and nutrients from the mother's blood diffuse through the villi to the baby's circulation, and carbon dioxide and waste products travel in the opposite direction into the maternal circulation.

Operating this continuous shuttle service between the two circulations is the placenta's most important function; but it also secretes many hormones and other biochemical messengers, including prostaglandins and factors affecting the clotting system, which enter the mother's bloodstream and reset her internal mechanisms to suit the requirements of pregnancy.

BLOOD CIRCULATION AND BLOOD PRESSURE

Pregnancy sets off profound changes in the workings of the mother's circulatory system, largely because of the need to divert extra blood to parts of the body concerned with supporting the pregnancy, including the kidneys, lungs, skin and breasts, as well as the uterus.

The circulation (Fig. 3.3)

Blood is distributed around the body via a closed system of blood vessels. An adult has about 5 litres (8 pints) of blood flowing around the system, propelled by the pumping action of the left side of the heart into arteries, which branch into progressively smaller vessels that terminate in microscopic capillaries, which reach every part of the body.

The walls of these capillaries are so thin that oxygen and nutrients diffuse through them to supply the surrounding tissues, while waste products, including carbon dioxide, pass from the tissues back to the blood. Blue, deoxygenated blood passed back into the capillaries drains into the veins, which return it to the right side of the heart,

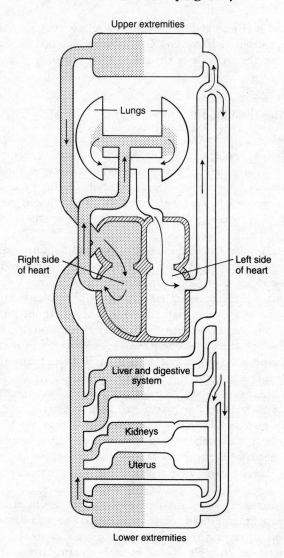

Fig. 3.3 Diagram of the heart and circulation. The left side of the heart distributes oxygenated blood to all parts of the body, through many arteries. Deoxygenated blood (stippled) returns to the right side of the heart, in the veins. The right side of the heart pumps blood to the lungs where it is reoxygenated, and from where it returns to the left side of the heart to re-circulate.

from where it is pumped to the lungs to release its carbon dioxide waste and receive fresh oxygen. Red, oxygenated blood returns from the lungs to the left side of the heart, and the whole cycle begins again.

Controlling the blood flow

The body controls the flow of blood to its various parts according to their needs. For example, after a meal the flow of blood to the stomach and intestines is boosted to aid digestion while the flow to other parts, such as the muscles, is reduced. During exercise, this process is reversed to favour the muscles. Blood flow is regulated by automatic processes, which constrict certain arteries and dilate others.

The flow of blood around the circulation is also influenced by the *heart rate*—the number of times the heart empties itself per minute —and the *stroke volume*—the amount of blood pumped out each time. Multiplying the heart rate by the stroke volume gives the total *cardiac output*, which is the volume of blood pumped from the heart each minute. The cardiac output varies according to need and, while the output at rest is about five litres per minute, during exertion or in extreme stress it can rise as high as 30 litres (more than 50 pints) per minute.

When the heart contracts (beats) it forces blood through the arteries under considerable pressure to keep it moving around the body. The pressure of blood within the arteries rises and falls with each heartbeat: the peak pressure, attained while the heart is contracting, is known as the *systolic pressure*; the lowest pressure, reached when the heart relaxes between beats, is known as the *diastolic pressure*.

Blood pressure plays a significant role in the health of an individual as abnormally high pressure—*hypertension*—can damage the circulation, increasing the risk of heart disease or stroke. This is why doctors check people's blood pressure, particularly as they get older.

Measuring blood pressure

Blood pressure is normally measured in the brachial artery, which supplies the forearm, using an instrument known as a *sphygmoman-ometer*. An inflatable cuff attached to a hand pump and a mercury pressure gauge is wrapped around the upper arm and inflated until the artery is squeezed shut. The doctor then slowly deflates the cuff and listens over the artery with a stethoscope: at first nothing can be heard, because the artery is shut and its wall is not vibrating, but as the air pressure in the cuff falls to below the peak pressure in the artery, the arterial wall begins to vibrate and a thumping sound can be heard as the blood forces its way past the obstructing cuff. The reading on the mercury pressure gauge at this point represents the systolic pressure. As the cuff deflates further the arterial sounds become muffled, and finally disappear when the cuff pressure falls to the level of the diastolic pressure.

A typical systolic blood pressure reading for a normal young person at rest is 110–120 millimetres of mercury (mmHg) and a typical diastolic reading is 70–80 mmHg. This would be written down as, say, 120/80 mmHg, and spoken of as '120 over 80'.

An individual's blood pressure is determined partly by the cardiac output and partly by resistance to flow in the arteries. This in turn depends on the quality both of the blood vessels and the blood itself: if the blood is thick or 'viscous' and the arteries tight and constricted the resistance to flow is high and it takes considerable pressure to force the blood through the arteries. But if the blood is optimally thin and the arteries relaxed and wide open, the resistance is low enough to keep even a high blood flow circulating at low pressure.

Blood pressure tends to rise with age, mainly because the arteries lose their elasticity, becoming more rigid, so a 'normal' blood pressure reading for a 60-year-old might be considered high for a young adult. There are no rigid norms for blood pressure at any age because average pressure varies from person to person, while for any individual the pressure tends to fluctuate according to factors like exercise, stress, hormonal changes, posture, and even the time of day. For example, during rest or sleep the heart rate slows, the arteries relax, and the blood pressure falls; during exercise or exertion the heart rate and its force of contraction increase, causing the blood pressure to rise. Thus, the blood pressure is not fixed or constant: it changes from minute to minute and hour to hour and it takes more than one reading to establish an individual's average blood pressure.

Hypotension

Some people have blood pressure that is consistently lower than 'normal' levels, although doctors tend not to worry about such chronic *hypotension* because it is associated with a reduced risk of circulatory disease.

Hypertension

Hypertension is diagnosed if a person's blood pressure is significantly and consistently raised above the normal range for the individual's age group. Doctors tend to worry more about the diastolic (lower) reading, because this is less likely than the systolic figure to vary according to the stress of the moment. But, as systolic and diastolic pressures tend to rise and fall together, either reading can be used to diagnose hypertension.

There are many causes of chronically high blood pressure, including kidney disease, hormonal disorders, and reactions to various drugs, medicines, and foods. But in most cases no cause is detectable and the person is said to be suffering from *essential hypertension*.

Many women think that pregnancy causes an inevitable rise in blood pressure. This is not true: in fact pregnant women normally experience a marked drop in blood pressure during the first trimester, with the pressure reaching its lowest point about halfway through the pregnancy, then gradually rising in the final weeks to reach prepregnant levels at around full term. This early fall in blood pressure is part of the overall circulatory adaptation to pregnancy, the purpose of which is to increase the blood supply to the organs and tissues most closely involved with supporting the pregnancy, particularly the placenta.

Increased circulatory needs during pregnancy

Although the blood pressure does not usually increase during pregnancy, the resting cardiac output—the amount of blood pumped from the heart each minute—increases by 30 per cent to about 6.5 litres per minute in the first 10 weeks and stays at this level until term. To achieve this increased output, the heart rate is stepped up by about 15 beats per minute and the volume of blood pumped with each stroke also rises. Increased cardiac output would normally raise the pressure in the arteries, but in pregnancy the opposite happens because the arteries relax and dilate under hormonal influences, greatly reducing the resistance to flow.

The major targets of this increased blood flow are the uterus, which nourishes the baby; the lungs and kidneys, which eliminate the baby's waste; the skin, which dissipates heat; and the breasts, in preparation for lactation.

To help cope with the increased circulatory needs of pregnancy, the mother's body makes more blood, partly by stepping up the production of red blood cells but mostly by boosting the volume of the plasma—the colourless liquid in which blood cells are suspended. This disproportionate increase in plasma volume means that the blood is more dilute than usual, with a lower concentration of red cells and haemoglobin, the red, iron-rich protein, which carries oxygen in red blood cells.

A progressive rise in plasma volume throughout pregnancy appears to be crucial to the success of a pregnancy, and large infants are linked with higher increases than small and growth-retarded babies.

CHANGES IN KIDNEY FUNCTION

The kidneys have the vital role of keeping body fluids in balance: this involves eliminating potentially poisonous waste substances and excess water and ensuring that useful nutrients are retained in the bloodstream. In pregnancy their function is greatly enhanced because they have to process an increased volume of fluids and eliminate extra waste from the baby.

The waste products generated in the body include urea (from proteins), creatinine (from muscles), and uric acid (from genetic materials). These substances pass out of the body's cells and are carried in the bloodstream to the kidneys, which are situated in the loins above the waist, one on either side of the spinal column. Here, the waste products are filtered out of the blood, along with any excess water, and turned into urine for excretion.

Filtering the blood

When blood is delivered to the kidney it first passes through one of more than a million tiny, sieve-like filtering units, called a *glomerulus* (plural *glomeruli*), which filters off plasma containing waste products and other small molecules. Proteins and other larger molecules do not normally pass through this filter and are retained in the bloodstream before being broken down in their turn into waste products.

The filtered plasma passes from the glomerulus into a long thin *tubule* surrounded by blood vessels. Here, further processing takes place, with useful small molecules, such as glucose and amino acids, being sucked back into the blood, and salts and water being partly reabsorbed to keep the blood concentration absolutely steady. Only waste products and excess water and mineral salts are retained in the tubule, which joins up with other tubules to conduct the urine out of the kidney into the ureter, and thence to the bladder. Each day the kidneys process about 170 litres of filtrate, of which only about one per cent is excreted as urine.

Impairment

Kidney function can be impaired for a number of reasons, including mechanical faults, infection, and damage caused by prolonged high blood pressure. Typical signs of impaired function are the retention of waste products in the blood and the appearance of blood, protein or other nutrients in the urine.

Changes during pregnancy

Pregnancy elicits dramatic improvements in kidney function. Blood flow to the kidneys is increased and the glomeruli carry out their filtering task at a faster rate. In consequence, waste products are excreted more efficiently than normal, and their concentrations in the blood are reduced.

The function of the tubules also changes in pregnancy. They lose some of their ability to reabsorb glucose and small proteins, so that small amounts leak out into the urine from time to time; but they reabsorb more sodium and water than usual, so that a reduced proportion of body fluids is excreted as urine.

Monitoring kidney function

Kidney function is monitored during pregnancy because departures from the norm can give early indication of complications, particularly pre-eclampsia. The most basic test is the dipstick urine test: this reveals the presence of protein, which should not be detectable in significant amounts if the kidneys are working properly. If a dipstick test gives an abnormal result, a more thorough assessment can be made by subjecting a urine sample collected over 24 hours to laboratory analysis.

Kidney function can also be monitored by means of blood tests to measure the concentration of waste products such as urea, creatinine, and uric acid. Abnormally high concentrations suggest impaired kidney function.

Why pregnant women swell

A vital function of the kidneys is to maintain the amount of water in body fluids at a constant level. That is why, on hot days, when we lose more water than usual in sweat, we pass a reduced volume of very concentrated urine. On the other hand, after drinking a large amount of fluid, we pass an increased volume of very dilute urine.

In pregnancy the body fluids become more dilute as more water than usual is retained in the body by the kidneys. Some of this excess water is stored in the tissues, particularly of the hands and feet, leading to the swelling (oedema), which is so typical of pregnancy. Most normal pregnant women develop some oedema in the last trimester; indeed there is good evidence that *some* oedema is more healthy than *no* oedema.

The cells of body tissues are embedded in a gelatinous mix of proteins called the *extracellular matrix*, which can retain fluid, rather like a sponge. This matrix appears to become more spongy than usual in pregnancy and holds on to more fluid. This effect is compounded by the fact that blood capillaries tend to become more permeable in pregnancy, allowing water to leak from the bloodstream into the tissues. Unfortunately, the normal, and indeed desirable, oedema of late pregnancy can be confused with more dramatic changes caused by pre-eclampsia, leading many healthy pregnant women to worry unduly. More of this in Chapter 4.

WHY BLOOD CLOTS MORE READILY IN PREGNANCY

The system that solidifies blood into clots to repair damaged and leaky blood vessels becomes more efficient in pregnancy; but this carries risks as well as benefits.

The circulatory system is a vast and complex network of blood vessels, all of which have the capacity to be damaged—even by relatively small injuries—and become leaky. Leaks may also develop during the ceaseless repair and remodelling activity, which affects the blood vessels as much as any other living structures. The risk of blood vessel damage is increased in pregnancy because of the intense circulatory activity around the placenta. The risk is particularly high immediately after delivery, when the placenta separates from the wall of the uterus, and the many arteries and veins carrying all the extra blood are suddenly severed.

The body deals with damaged blood vessels and contains the consequent leakage of blood by solidifying blood into solid clots as and when required. This activity has to be precisely controlled because inadequate clotting could enable a mere pinprick injury to bleed indefinitely, while excessive clotting could block a blood vessel completely, causing damage to whatever organ it supplies.

Blood clots are formed by interaction between two components of blood—*fibrin*, which forms the 'cement' of the clot; and *platelets*, which form the 'brickwork'. When a blood vessel springs a leak, the soluble blood protein, *fibrinogen*, is converted with explosive speed to insoluble fibrin, which at first is soft and weak, like newly-mixed cement, but rapidly hardens and strengthens.

Platelets

The production of fibrin activates the platelets—small specialized blood cells, which are loaded with potent proteins and other chemicals. Activated platelets stick together and embed themselves in fibrin to build up the solid body of a blood clot, at the same time summoning more platelets to the site of the injury and stimulating the production of additional fibrin. Platelets release substances that cause the leaking vessel to go into spasm, so effectively providing its own tourniquet; they also attract specialized cells to the site to tidy up and repair the damage. So even as the leak is plugged, reconstruction is under way.

Platelets are produced in large quantities; there are about 350 000 in every millimetre of blood. As they have a short life, of about 10–14 days, the supply needs to be constantly replenished. Clearly, these platelets are very potent and busy cells and, as they also play an important role in the genesis of pre-eclampsia, they will appear again in Chapter 4.

Maintaining a healthy balance

As mentioned above, a delicate balance must be struck between keeping the blood fluid enough to ferry oxygen and nutrients around the body and maintaining an efficient clotting system. The body achieves this balance by countering a powerful clotting tendency with equally powerful mechanisms that suppress unnecessary clotting.

In pregnancy, this balance is reset, so that the clotting system responds more briskly and at a lower threshold to activation cues. This is partly achieved through an increase in the blood concentration of fibrinogen, which makes the fibrin cement.

The underlying purpose of this change must be to reduce the hazards of bleeding in pregnancy and childbirth. But the price of this protection is an increased risk of inappropriate clotting, which can block important blood vessels and lead to dangerous complications like pulmonary embolism.

Platelets are busier than usual during pregnancy and, because they die after performing their tasks—like bees after stinging—it is common to find a slightly lower than normal concentration in the blood, although more than enough for good health. A very marked fall in the platelet count, as sometimes happens with pre-eclampsia, is a serious sign because it poses the risk of complete breakdown of the clotting system, giving rise to uncontrollable bleeding.

FEEDING THE UNBORN BABY

Pregnancy triggers off important changes in the way the body processes food, enabling the growing baby to make the maximum use of whatever nourishment is available. For example, some nutrients, particularly the iron that is needed to boost the mother's blood volume and build the baby's circulation, are absorbed more efficiently than usual from food, and the maternal blood levels of many other nutrients, including protein, folic acid, and vitamin B12, are altered in a way that is thought to favour delivery to the baby rather than the mother. At the same time, the baby itself operates as a highly efficient parasite, plundering the mother's blood for the nutrients it needs and ensuring that deficiencies affect her health before its own.

The baby's agent in this operation is the placenta, which has the ability to condense nutrients, particularly vitamins, for the benefit of the baby, so that their concentrations in cord and fetal blood may be five or even ten times greater than in the mother's bloodstream, particularly towards the end of the pregnancy.

Maternal nutrition

A pregnant woman's body also has the facility to slow down the rate at which energy from food is used, so that more than usual is conserved to maintain the growing baby and all its supporting tissues and to store extra fat in preparation for breastfeeding.

Studies of women in rural Africa have revealed a significant slowing in the metabolic rate in early pregnancy, sometimes persisting until the start of the third trimester. This could be explained as Nature's way of protecting pregnant women and their babies from the effects of famine and enabling them to maintain their pregnancies on a low food intake. But such metabolic adjustments are not confined to women in developing countries—similar changes have been noted in a group of well-fed British women, studied before and during pregnancy. This study, by the Medical Research Council's Dunn Nutrition Unit, in Cambridge, revealed an astonishing amount of variation between individuals. While some showed a marked *reduction* in their resting metabolic rate in the first two trimesters, others showed an *increase*. Significantly, though, the thin women in the study tended to be the slow burners of energy, implying that Nature's purpose is to counteract the effects of food shortage. This is one of many recent findings that have helped to bury the Victorian theory that pregnant women need to 'eat for two' to produce healthy, well-grown babies.

Even the moderate recommendation from the Department of Health that pregnant women need an extra 200 calories per day, taking their total daily intake to 2400 calories, is now considered outdated by most experts, as women have been shown to produce babies of good weight on much lower intakes. For example, nutritionists from the London School of Hygiene and Tropical Medicine, who examined the diets of more than 250 women from London and Edinburgh at intervals throughout pregnancy, found they all produced healthy babies on average daily intakes of 2000–2200 calories.

The quality of nutrition

But if the *quantity* of food eaten in pregnancy is less important than has previously been suggested, can the *quality* of a pregnant woman's diet affect the outcome of her pregnancy? The latest research suggests that it can. In a study on the relationship between maternal nutrition and birth weight, carried out by scientists from the Nuffield Laboratories of Comparative Medicine, attached to London Zoo, more than 400 women were asked to keep a diary of all food and drink they consumed during one week in the first trimester of pregnancy; their food diaries were later correlated with the birth weights of their babies.

The study revealed that mothers whose babies weighed 3 kg (6.6 lb) or less had recorded lower intakes of almost all nutrients than the mothers of heavier babies. The nutrients most significantly associated with birth weight were the B group of vitamins, sodium, chloride, magnesium, phosphorus, and iron. In a separate study by the same authors, low intakes of a number of nutrients during pregnancy, particularly those nutrients found in high-fibre foods, were shown to be associated with reduced head circumference at birth—this measurement being an indicator of brain development.

At first reading, these findings appear to contradict our previous statement that the baby, being a parasite, plunders nutrients *ad lib* from its mother's bloodstream. However, the placenta, which scavenges on the baby's behalf, is not fully established until the end of the first trimester; so a poor diet in the preconception period and the early weeks of pregnancy could have an adverse effect on the baby.

The implication that it is what you eat in very early pregnancy that counts was reinforced by a further finding of the Nuffield scientists that vitamin and mineral supplementation in the last two trimesters of pregnancy had no significant effect on average birth weight.

Two general points

It is not the purpose of this book to set down an optimal diet for pregnancy. Our aim in this chapter is to create a better understanding of what goes wrong in pre-eclampsia by looking at the various ways in which the mother's body adapts to pregnancy. Later in the book (see Chapter 6) we will concentrate on the various theories about how diet may contribute to the evolution of pre-eclampsia and what you can do about it. However, two general points about diet in pregnancy should be clear from what we have said so far:

1. Pregnant women need to think about their diet in terms of quality rather than quantity, which, in broad terms, means maximizing intake of fresh whole foods, including cereals, fruit, vegetables, fish, and lean meat and minimizing consumption of refined foods high in fats and sugars.

2. The time to improve the quality of the diet is before conception, so that the early embryo is well provided for in the weeks before the placenta is established.

Sickness

Where does this leave women who are bedevilled by the sickness that is so common in early pregnancy? Major nutritional deficiencies can sometimes arise as a result of severe vomiting (hyperemesis) and this can, although very rarely, lead to serious weight loss and even maternal death. The milder sickness, which is suffered by nearly three-quarters of women in early pregnancy, has not been shown to affect birth weight. Many women, in any case, find that eating actually relieves their nausea, and for them the trick is to resort to healthy foods rather than high-calorie snacks to quell their symptoms. But even those who can't stomach much food at all during this difficult time should, if their original diet was healthy, have reserves of nutrients that their babies can draw on until a normal eating pattern is re-established.

THE SIGNIFICANCE OF WEIGHT GAIN

Weight gain in pregnancy is an emotive and confusing subject, particularly in connection with pre-eclampsia. It used to be very common for doctors to set strict limits on how much weight their patients were allowed to gain, mostly because sudden, dramatic weight gain carries an increased risk of pre-eclampsia. However, it is now known that this weight gain is a sign of fluid retention, not over-eating and that it is a *consequence*, not a *cause*, of pre-eclampsia. So no pregnant woman should be misled into thinking that keeping her weight down will reduce her risk of suffering the disease. In fact, doctors are now less prescriptive in general about weight gain in pregnancy because it is recognized that some women need to gain more weight than others and can do so with no lasting effects, and also that weight gain in pregnancy has very little bearing on birth weight.

The average weight gain in pregnancy is 24–28 lb although one textbook, *Clinical Physiology in Obstetrics* (edited by Frank Hytten and Geoffrey Chamberlain, Blackwell Scientific Publications, 1980) points out that healthy women with normal pregnancies may gain no weight at all at one extreme and as much as twice the average at the other.

A major study of more than 16 000 pregnant women, carried out in the US in the 1970s, showed that light women eat more and gain more weight than heavier ones. The same conclusion emerged from a subsequent German study of almost 8000 pregnant women.

Most of the weight gained in pregnancy is due to an increase in maternal rather than fetal tissue, including the enlarged uterus and breasts, the expanded blood volume, and the extra body water. It also includes an extra 3.5 kg (7.7 lb) or so of fat, which is stored in midpregnancy to buffer mother and baby against the effects of food shortage in the last trimester and provide a reserve of calories for breast-feeding. This fat store appears to be laid down automatically, regardless of how much the mother eats.

After delivery, a mother can expect her excess weight to be the sum of this fat store plus whatever she has gained through over-eating. Fluid retention can account for substantial weight gain, but is rapidly lost after delivery. The fat store is normally dissipated during breast-feeding; women who choose to bottle-feed may need to diet to lose it.

LANDMARKS IN FETAL GROWTH AND DEVELOPMENT

Fetal development proceeds at an astonishing rate in the 12 weeks following conception and by the end of this time the baby has assumed a recognizable shape, with face and features, limbs, extremities, and all the major internal organs.

By 14 weeks of pregnancy the baby is completely formed and the placenta is fully established. From then on the emphasis is on growth and maturation. Fetal growth is continuous from conception onwards, although the rate of growth progressively flattens out as the pregnancy advances. The average birth weight of full-term babies in England is 3.3 kg (7.3 lb), and any baby weighing less than 2.5 kg (5.5 lb) is said to be of low birth weight.

Birth weight

A baby's birth weight at term is affected by many different factors, most of which are predetermined. These include:

- *Maternal size*: heavy and/or tall women tend to have heavier babies than light and/or short women, regardless of their partners' size;

- *Sex*: boys are slightly heavier than girls;

- *Maternal age*: young women tend to have the lightest babies;

- *Birth order*: each sibling tends to be heavier than the one before;

- *Maternal nutrition*: women on extremely poor diets tend to have small babies, although the converse is not true;

- *Congenital defects and infections*: these are associated with small babies;

- *Maternal habits*: cigarette smoking, heavy drinking, and drug abuse are all linked with low birth weight;

- *Maternal illness*: diabetic women tend to produce extra-large babies while pre-eclampsia is associated with low birth weight.

Low birth weight

Low birth weight is a major health risk. Over two-thirds of UK babies who die in the perinatal period weigh less than 2.5 kg at birth. Most of these babies are small because they are premature, but a minority are small despite being mature. Of these 'small-for-dates' babies, some are smaller than average for genetic reasons and are perfectly healthy, but others are small because they did not grow well in the womb. These babies, said to suffer from *intrauterine growth retardation* (IUGR), are at special risk both before and after birth.

Identification of low birthweight babies

Doctors use population norms known as 'percentiles' to help identify babies with growth problems during pregnancy. Those that are lighter than the 10th percentile—meaning that they are smaller than 90 per cent of babies of the same maturity—are generally considered small-for-dates and are monitored carefully for signs of distress, which might point to the need for early delivery. This risk-rating system is not foolproof as it includes many babies who are genetically small and excludes others who are growth-retarded despite being heavier than the 10th percentile.

Monitoring fetal growth

Fetal growth can be monitored in two ways: by manual measurement and, with considerably greater accuracy, by ultrasound scanning.

Manual examination

Before the 1970s the only way to estimate the size of an unborn child was to 'feel' the mother's abdomen externally. A skilled doctor or midwife could get some idea of what was going on, but the technique was and is notoriously unreliable: most small-for-dates babies were simply not detected.

The accuracy of manual examination has been improved to some extent by using tape measurements of the expanding uterus. First the top (*fundus*) of the womb is identified and then the distance from here to the front of the bony pelvis is measured. Conveniently, this distance, measured in centimetres, should correspond to the maturity of the baby, so that at 28 weeks, for example, the uterus should measure about 28 cm from top to bottom. If the measurement is 4 cm or more short of what it should be, there is an increased risk that the baby is small-for-dates. This method has its own inaccuracies: the size of the uterus will not necessarily correspond to the maturity of the baby if, for example, there is a large volume of amniotic fluid, if the mother is carrying twins or if the baby's head has already 'engaged' in the pelvis. If the mother is very overweight, it may be difficult to locate the fundus in the first place.

Ultrasound

Given the uncertainties of manual examination, the introduction of ultrasound scanning was a giant leap forward. Scanning offers reliable information about the size and growth rate of a baby because the dimensions of the head, the girth of the abdomen, and the length of particular bones can be monitored with remarkable accuracy.

It is normal practice for a 'dating' scan to be carried out early in the second trimester, when the maturity of the baby can be pinpointed precisely by measuring the diameter between its temples (biparietal diameter, or BPD); this and other dimensions can then be used as 'baseline' measurements if further scans are needed.

A series of scans are needed for a really clear idea of how well or otherwise a baby is growing. The measurements can be plotted on charts, which also show average growth curves and the range of normal values for each stage of pregnancy. Obviously, serial scanning is carried out only in cases where there is a real risk of growth retardation.

Normal growth is a crucial measure of fetal well-being, but there are also other pointers:

Fetal movement

The growing baby begins to move as soon as its muscles have developed in the first trimester, but the mother is unaware of this activity until the uterus is sufficiently stretched for the movements to be felt against the abdominal wall, usually between 16 and 20 weeks of pregnancy. The movements start as vague flutterings, becoming stronger and more persistent day by day until they are felt as thumping or kicking sensations. The most powerful movements are usually felt between 30 and 32 weeks, when the baby is very strong and still has plenty of room to manoeuvre. In the last 2 weeks, when space in the womb is restricted, the movements may change from kicking to squirming.

An active baby is a well baby, as every pregnant woman instinctively recognizes, which is why doctors tend to ask how well the baby is moving at antenatal checks. There is no 'right' number of daily movements, but it may be significant if a baby who normally moves frequently and vigorously becomes unusually quiet and still.

In the last few months of pregnancy, babies begin to develop patterns of alternating rest and activity, with quiet periods lasting on average about 20 minutes and rarely longer than 40 or 50. There is also a 24-hour cycle, with babies tending to be most active late at night or very early in the morning.

'Kick charts' compiled by mothers are often used as a screening process in the last trimester if there is some concern about the baby's well-being. The mother is asked to count the number of separate fetal movements in a specified period of time and contact the hospital if they don't conform to a given norm, such as 10 movements in 12 hours.

However, not all movements are noticed by mothers, particularly if there is a lot of amniotic fluid or if the placenta is lying in front of the baby, and the natural variations in fetal movement are wide enough to make any 'norms' slightly suspect. So while it may be reassuring for a mother to get a 'normal' result, most 'low counts' turn out to be false alarms.

Fetal breathing

The baby has to learn to use all his or her muscles before birth, including the diaphragm and respiratory muscles, which will be used for breathing after birth. These 'practice' breathing movements can be detected by ultrasound scanning, particularly in the last trimester, and are a sign that all is well. The movements are rarely continuous and may not take place at all in any given 10–15 minute period, but it would be very unusual for no breathing to occur over half an hour.

Fetal heart rate

The baby's heartbeat is, of course, the ultimate sign of life. With sensitive ultrasound equipment it can be discerned within 4 weeks of conception, and in the second half of pregnancy can be easily heard through an ear trumpet.

While the *presence* of the heartbeat proves the baby is alive, the *pattern* of that heartbeat, recorded over 30–60 minutes, can provide more subtle information about the baby's state of health. The fetal heart runs about twice as fast as the adult heart, although it slows a little as the baby matures in the womb. However, the heart does not beat at a fixed rate but fluctuates second by second and minute by minute, according to impulses transmitted by the brain. This means that under normal circumstances the interval between each heartbeat varies slightly so that the baseline rate is never totally flat, even when the baby is sleeping.

This 'variability' is a sign of healthy brain activity and is particularly marked when the baby is wakeful and active: with each movement the heart rate accelerates by 15–40 beats per minute. Doctors used to believe these accelerations represented a reaction to the movements and referred to the typical pattern as a 'reactive heart trace' but it is now known that both movement and accelerations are separate, independent responses to a busy, active brain.

About once every hour or so, the baby's brain has a rest when it slips into deep sleep. These periods are characterized by few movements and no accelerations in the heart rate. In the past doctors misread this temporary lack of activity as a sign of abnormality, but its significance is now better understood.

The baby's heart rate is sensitive to any problem affecting brain activity, including shortage of oxygen. For this reason heart rate monitoring by means of *cardiotocography* (CTG) has become a standard technique when problems are suspected. CTG monitors use ultrasound techniques to record fetal movements and the heart rate pattern, while a separate device records any uterine activity. This is important because the 'tightenings' known as *Braxton Hicks contractions* cause transient oxygen deprivation if the blood supply to the baby is inadequate, and this is reflected in abnormalities of the heart rate.

Amniotic fluid volume

The unborn baby floats in a fluid-filled cavity encircled by a very fine membrane known as the *amnion*. The amniotic fluid cushions and protects the baby, allowing it to move freely and grow without restraint, and is essential for normal lung development.

Problems can arise if there is either too much (*polyhydramnios*) or too little (*oligohydramnios*) fluid in the cavity. Oligohydramnios, which is detectable by ultrasound scan, is associated with growth retardation while polyhydramnios, which is usually obvious because it causes gross abdominal distension, poses the risk of premature labour or rupture of the membranes. Oligohydramnios is sometimes a sign of pre-eclampsia. Polyhydramnios can also be associated with pre-eclampsia but is more commonly a complication of twin or diabetic pregnancy.

Thanks to modern technology, the world inside the womb is now much less of a mystery than it was 20 years ago and surprisingly precise assessments can be made of potential problems.

BLOOD FLOW AND THE HEALTHY PLACENTA

Everything needed for the baby's growth and maturation, including oxygen, protein, carbohydrate, fatty acids, vitamins, and minerals, must travel in the mother's bloodstream to the placenta before they can be delivered to the baby via the umbilical vein.

Antibodies, giving the baby resistance to certain infections for some time after birth, reach the baby in the same way and so, in a less welcome fashion, do alcohol; nicotine; a few infective organisms, such as rubella and listeria; and a range of drugs. Waste products generated by the baby travel in the opposite direction, delivered to the placenta via the umbilical arteries to be absorbed into the mother's circulation and excreted by her lungs and kidneys.

The placenta is fully functional from the beginning of the second trimester but to keep pace with the baby's demands it must grow in tandem with the baby. The size of a full-term placenta is directly linked to the baby's size and it tips the scales at about one-sixth of the baby's weight.

As the placenta grows with the pregnancy, the chorionic villi— those 'leaves' of the placental tree across which exchange of oxygen and nutrients takes place—multiply and mature, becoming smaller but more numerous. At the same time their outer trophoblast coating thins while the inner fetal blood vessels dilate; these changes ensure that the placenta works with increasing efficiency to meet the baby's ever-growing needs.

A range of fetal problems, including pre-eclampsia, growth retardation, and even intrauterine death are sometimes ascribed to 'placental insufficiency'—a term that implies that the placenta itself may fail to meet the baby's demands. In fact, the placenta rarely becomes insufficient because of its own inherent limitations: it has considerable reserves and can withstand the loss of 30–40 per cent of its villi without any evidence of declining performance. But what *has* become increasingly clear is that the placenta can become insufficient as a result of external problems; and the common factor in most cases is reduced maternal blood flow due to inadequate dilation of the spiral arteries feeding the placenta.

Assessing placental blood flow

Doctors are now able to assess the adequacy of placental blood flow by means of a special ultrasound technique known as 'Doppler' scanning, which analyses the speed of flow through blood vessels. Almost any artery in the body can be studied with Doppler equipment, but in maternity units it is most commonly used to examine the flow through one of the arteries in the umbilical cord.

Essentially, the test reveals whether or not the baby's side of the circulation is working well. The flow of blood through the cord should be continuous, accelerating with each fetal heartbeat. If the flow is intermittent, moving when the heart beats but stopping in between beats, the supply line to the baby is under threat. A poor Doppler result does not mean the baby is in immediate trouble but, as restricted blood flow is usually a progressive problem, it does suggest that early delivery will be necessary at some stage.

HOW LABOUR AFFECTS MOTHER AND BABY

Labour poses a stiffer challenge to the reserves of both mother and baby than either have faced in pregnancy. A well mother and baby linked by a fully functional placenta should weather the trial, as long as labour is not impeded by mechanical difficulties. But latent problems that may have remained unsuspected in pregnancy are likely to be revealed by labour.

The challenge to the mother

On the mother's side, the anxiety, pain, and sheer hard work of labour tend to push up the blood pressure. Sometimes the first signs of pre-eclampsia appear in labour, and it is also a classic time for a first eclamptic fit. Women with blood pressure problems are often advised to take their pain relief in the form of epidural anaesthesia, which numbs the lower half of the body; it also provokes a number of changes in the circulatory system, which work together to reduce blood pressure. General anaesthesia, which is often used for emergency Caesarean sections, also tends to reduce the blood pressure, although the initial *intubation* procedure, which allows the mother's lungs to be ventilated during the operation, causes an intense rise in blood pressure for some 60–90 seconds. For this reason, anaesthetists prefer to avoid general anaesthesia for hypertensive women, although there is little evidence that it does any real harm.

The drug syntometrine is usually given by injection immediately after delivery of the baby's head to induce intense uterine contractions, which will hasten the delivery of the placenta and so reduce the risk of postpartum haemorrhage. One component of this drug, ergometrine, also causes the arteries to contract, which tends to raise the blood pressure, particularly in women who are prone to hypertension. Some doctors therefore prefer to incur the slight risk of haemorrhage rather than provoke dangerously heightened blood pressures in women with pre-eclampsia.

The challenge to the baby

Labour challenges the baby largely through the stress it imposes on the placenta. The force of each contraction temporarily obstructs blood flow to the placenta and, while a healthy placenta has the reserves to make up the delivery of oxygen to the baby between contractions, a placenta compromised by long-standing restriction of its blood supply does not, and the resultant oxygen shortage causes fetal distress, which calls for urgent delivery. The main sign of fetal distress during labour is a dramatic change in the pattern of the heart rate, sometimes coupled with the passage of meconium—the thick green substance which is normally held in the baby's rectum until after delivery—out of the vagina. It is standard practice to screen for fetal distress by monitoring the heart rate at regular intervals during labour; in high-risk cases the monitoring is often continuous. The heart rate can be monitored externally by ultrasound or, more directly, by passing a lead from a monitor through the cervix and attaching it to the baby's scalp. More direct evidence of oxygen shortage can be sought by analysing a few drops of blood from the baby's scalp. If the baby is in distress the acid levels in its blood will be high, and this calls for prompt delivery.

BACK TO NORMAL AGAIN

Except for the changes relating to breast-feeding, all the many maternal adaptations to pregnancy, which have developed over 9 months, suddenly become redundant after delivery. What follows is a period of tumultuous change as the body strives to restore the order of the prepregnant state.

The most dramatic changes take place in the first week, when the uterus rapidly shrinks within the pelvis, the reproductive tract springs back into shape, hormone levels fall and excess fluid is lost. After the first week, the return to normality continues at a much slower pace. The postnatal period, or puerperium, traditionally lasts 6 weeks, but it can take considerably longer for all the adaptations of pregnancy to be reversed. Indeed some changes, including stretch marks, darker pigmentation of the nipples and abdomen, and enlargement of the uterus, are permanent.

The circulation

Restoration of normal circulation is a particularly complex business. By the end of pregnancy, the spiral arteries, which supply the placenta, have expanded to carry about 100 times more blood than usual. Once the placenta has been delivered this part of the circulation is suddenly extinguished and although some of the blood flowing to this area is lost at delivery, most of it is squeezed back into the general circulation in a sudden surge, which imposes considerable strain on the system and forces the heart to work harder for a day or so.

It takes a few days for the body to reduce the volume of circulating blood to prepregnant levels. Water accounted for most of the additional volume in pregnancy and it is mostly water that is shed after delivery, enabling the blood to regain its previous concentrations of red cells, haemoglobin and other constituents. Although the restoration of normal blood volume is rapid, the cardiac output takes several weeks to fall to prepregnant levels because, although the heart rate rapidly returns to normal, the stroke volume remains elevated for some time.

Platelets

We have already described how platelets are slightly reduced in pregnancy, and more so with pre-eclampsia. In the first 2 days after delivery it is normal for the platelet count to drop still further, but this is followed by a surge of fresh platelets into the circulation and a rapid rise in the platelet count, which remains elevated for some weeks. Consequently the blood is more 'clottable' than usual, which explains the increased risk of dangerous, obstructive clotting (*thrombosis*) in the postnatal period.

Blood pressure

Curiously, many women whose blood pressures have remained normal throughout pregnancy and labour become mildly hypertensive in the first few days after delivery. No-one is quite sure why this happens; in some cases it is because late pre-eclampsia has been suddenly triggered by labour; but in others it seems as if the sudden loss of factors that have helped to lower the blood pressure in pregnancy cause a temporary overshoot before the body regains its equilibrium.

Women who have suffered pre-eclampsia in pregnancy often remain hypertensive for a few weeks after delivery, although in most cases the blood pressure returns to normal by the end of the postnatal period.

4 · When things go wrong

At a routine antenatal test at 34 weeks, my blood pressure was raised, my fingers and legs were swollen and I had gained a lot of weight; in fact, I had put on a total of 22 kg—about 3½ stone—since the beginning of my pregnancy.

I was advised to rest at home and return to the clinic in a week's time. However, despite resting, the swelling did not go down and my blood pressure remained high, and on my last routine visit to the hospital, when it reached 170/115, I was admitted. After 2 days in hospital my blood pressure could only be controlled by injections and there were two 'plusses' of protein in my urine.

I was kept in hospital for 3 days before induction. I did not suffer fits, but on the morning of my induction my blood pressure was at first too high for them to proceed and I had the worst headache I've experienced in my life.

I didn't feel ill when I was admitted and needed some convincing that I was not going home. It was only when I was told that my placenta was failing that I realized how serious things were. I was delivered at 37 weeks by Caesarean section after the induction failed. My son weighed 6 lb 2 oz, but needed special care for 2 days as he had a low blood sugar level. I recovered very quickly, and on the fifth day we both went home.

Pat Hall

This was a classic case of severe pre-eclampsia; raised blood pressure and swelling in late pregnancy, followed by the appearance of protein in the urine and then by symptoms of illness, nipped in the bud by early delivery. But this is not the whole story—not by any means!

Pre-eclampsia was dubbed 'the disease of theories' by the German physician Zweifel in 1895. But it could be described just as aptly as 'the disease of exceptions'. There *is* a classic pattern, but there are too many exceptions to prove any overriding rule.

Pre-eclampsia normally shows itself in the third trimester of pregnancy, but it can appear at 20 weeks, or even earlier, or as late as several days after delivery. Overt illness is usually preceded by symptomless clinical signs, which can be detected in routine antenatal checks, but some women become suddenly and seriously ill without warning. High blood pressure and oedema are characteristic but not universal; women are most vulnerable in their first pregnancies but some suffer pre-eclampsia for the first time in a second or later pregnancy. Pre-eclampsia does not usually recur, although it can do sometimes, and the recurrence may be as severe or even worse than the first attack.

The chameleon-like mutability of this disease helps to explain why, despite being such a common complication of pregnancy, pre-eclampsia is so poorly understood, not merely by the women who suffer it but by the GPs, midwives and even specialist obstetricians who treat it.

Although the main underlying purpose of the regular antenatal checks offered to all pregnant women is to detect the earliest warning signs of pre-eclampsia, doctors and midwives continue to make mistakes in diagnosis when they are confronted with cases that do not fit the typical pattern. Their problems are compounded by the fact that the cause of pre-eclampsia is still unknown. This makes it impossible to use a standard diagnostic test, which would leave no room for the doubts and misconceptions that currently muddy the waters.

The most common misconception about pre-eclampsia is that it is essentially a disease of high blood pressure; this gives rise to the equally mistaken belief that if the blood pressure can somehow be prevented from rising or controlled once it has risen then the disease itself can be prevented or cured. In fact, high blood pressure and pre-eclampsia are not synonymous; neither is pre-eclampsia *caused* by high blood pressure and, although most people with pre-eclampsia do have raised blood pressure, this is not invariable.

Pre-eclampsia is much more than a circulatory disorder. It can affect and damage the mother's kidneys, liver, brain, eyes, blood clotting and nervous systems. It also affects the unborn baby, causing malnutrition, oxygen starvation and, in extreme cases, death *in utero*.

No-one knows the fundamental cause of this broad range of problems or why some women are more susceptible than others, although pre-eclampsia is known to run in families (see p. 88). It is also known that pre-eclamptic disturbances in both mother and baby are linked with problems in the placenta, and experts are increasingly inclined to view the whole condition as a 'sick placenta syndrome'.

Quite apart from the direct scientific evidence of placental involvement in pre-eclampsia, there are good logical reasons for believing that the disease must emanate from the placenta. First, pre-eclampsia only ever occurs during pregnancy or immediately after delivery; secondly, it is always cured by delivery; thirdly, and most significantly, women can suffer pre-eclampsia without having a baby in the womb—it is a known risk for women suffering from a rare complication of pregnancy called hydatidiform mole, when the development of the fertilized egg is so abnormal that an excessively large placenta develops without a fetus.

In summary: (i) you need to be pregnant to get pre-eclampsia; (ii) you need to have a placenta—but not necessarily a baby; and (iii) you can expect to recover once the placenta has been removed. All reasons why the disease can be deemed to originate in the placenta.

THE PROBLEM OF THE 'SICK PLACENTA'

What is going on inside the pre-eclamptic placenta? Why is it sick? The problem seems to arise from an inadequate supply of blood from the mother. As explained in the last chapter, blood is delivered to the placenta by numerous small 'spiral arteries', which are remodelled by embryonic cells in early pregnancy so that they can dilate to many times their normal size in order to carry a hugely increased volume of blood.

In pre-eclampsia, this remodelling process, which takes place between 6 and 18 weeks of pregnancy, is only partially successful, so that the spiral arteries remain relatively small-bored and thick-walled instead of becoming dilated and thin-walled. As a result, they are constitutionally unable to carry the greatly increased blood supply that the placenta will need later in pregnancy.

Ischaemia

During the second half of pregnancy the placenta continues to grow to meet the baby's ever-increasing demands. As it grows, it calls on the spiral arteries to deliver more and more blood from the mother. If these arteries are much narrower than they should be, there inevitably comes a time when supply can no longer match demand. The placenta begins to be short of blood (*ischaemic*) and from then on has to struggle to do its job without the necessary resources.

This blood shortage is compounded by a further problem affecting the spiral arteries. For some reason placental ischaemia triggers off a process called *acute atherosis*, in which a mixture of clotted blood, platelets, and fat-filled cells (lipophages) accumulates on the inner walls of these vital vessels. This furs-up the arteries and reduces their blood-bearing capacity still further. So a bad situation is made worse and the ischaemic placenta is even more lacking in blood.

Scientific evidence of ischaemia

Scientists have found direct evidence of these changes when examining the placentas of pre-eclamptic women after delivery. Under a microscope it is possible to see the consequences of ischaemia, most notably areas of the placenta that have been so deprived of oxygen that the tissue has died. This does not damage the baby directly but, with parts of the placenta destroyed, the baby has to cope with a damaged and inefficient supply line.

The effects of ischaemia on the mother

How does this placental problem lead to illness in the mother? This is easier to understand if you recall from Chapter 3 the profound and wide-ranging adaptations the mother's body has to make in pregnancy, all of which are stimulated by the placenta and its membranes. The healthy placenta is like the conductor of a large and intricate piece of orchestral music—the harmonious and balanced progression of pregnancy, which is so essential for a successful outcome, depends on the many different signals and messages it gives out. A sick placenta, starved of oxygen, conducts the piece wrong: the orchestration of pregnancy becomes discordant and unbalanced, and the mother suffers as well as the baby.

This outline of the placenta's role in causing pre-eclampsia must be considered provisional. There is still much to be learned before it can be said to be proved beyond all doubt. What we *can* say is that the theory of the sick placenta fits what is known about the disease and is supported by experimental evidence. Pre-eclampsia does not occur in most animals, although something like it can be induced if the placental blood supply is artificially restricted.

What scientists are unsure of is the nature of the signals coming from the sick placenta that make a woman's blood pressure rise, cause her to retain fluid, leak protein into her urine, and so on.

Neither do they understand the root cause of the problem—
what it is that hinders the crucial transformation of the spiral
arteries.

The ideas presented so far have some very important implications
for our understanding of the disease. The first, as already mentioned,
is that high blood pressure is not fundamental to pre-eclampsia but
simply one of its many effects.

The second is that pre-eclampsia can affect a baby as much as its
mother. Most women, and indeed many doctors, think of pre-
eclampsia as a maternal illness in which the baby is accidentally
involved. But in fact it is a *shared* illness. Modern technology proves
this to be true. Until quite recently the baby was a mysterious and
almost unknowable part of pregnancy, at least as far as doctors and
midwives were concerned. But now they can 'see' with ultrasound
scanning the extent to which the baby suffers as the placenta gets
more and more ischaemic.

The baby's problems are different from the mother's: they do
not, for example, include high blood pressure or proteinuria. But
changes affecting the baby, such as slowing of the rate of growth,
are as important a sign of a sick placenta as these more familiar
maternal changes.

Sometimes the problems of the baby are more prominent and
urgent than those of its mother; sometimes the opposite is true. But
both are involved because the primary disorder is in the organ that
joins them—the placenta.

A THREE-STAGE DISEASE

The theory of the sick placenta offers a useful way of thinking about
how pre-eclampsia develops. There are three distinct stages of the
disease, which follow each other in a chronological sequence:

- *Stage 1* is the invisible placental disorder.

- *Stage 2* consists of detectable but largely symptomless changes in
  mother and baby as their bodies strive to adapt to and compensate
  for the sick placenta.

- *Stage 3*, which should be preventable by prompt diagnosis and
  action in the second stage, is serious, potentially life-threatening
  illness in mother and/or baby.

The first stage is set in motion in the first half of pregnancy, when the placental blood flow is being established. The second stage does not normally begin to develop until the second half of pregnancy. The third stage is less predictable—it can follow as early as days, or even hours, or as late as weeks after the onset of the second stage.

The effect of a sick placenta on an unborn baby is self-evident: the baby is totally dependent on the placenta to transport oxygen and nutrients from the mother's circulation to its own and a sick placenta offers an inadequate supply line, with slow but increasing deprivation of oxygen and food. The earliest detectable sign of pre-eclampsia in the baby is slower-than-expected growth, as revealed by manual examination or ultrasound scanning.

The image of the placenta as a conductor (p. 57) is a useful aid to understanding its effects on the mother. In a normal pregnancy, the healthy placenta orchestrates a variety of changes for the benefit of mother and baby, including expanded blood volume, enhanced kidney function, and a brisker blood clotting response. In a pre-eclamptic pregnancy, the sick placenta destabilizes a range of maternal functions to the detriment of mother and baby.

Second-stage illness

The most important signs of second-stage disease in the mother are raised blood pressure, protein in the urine and sudden, dramatic swelling. These changes fall short of actual illness, and most women who display them feel perfectly well. This fact is one of the most important 'catches' about pre-eclampsia. It is very hard for a woman —and even for her doctor—to accept that a major problem is brewing when she feels and looks so well.

The second stage for both mother and baby is a balancing act; the individual systems of the body can only tolerate so much disturbance before they begin to break down or go out of control. What gives way and how soon varies from pregnancy to pregnancy, but the result is always serious illness—the third stage of pre-eclampsia.

Third-stage illness

Third-stage illness can prove rapidly fatal for mother or baby, but fortunately most cases of pre-eclampsia never get that far because antenatal care is geared towards detecting it in its second stage, while the problem is still contained, so that serious complications can be pre-empted by early delivery.

The remainder of this chapter takes a closer look at the manifestations of pre-eclampsia in both mother and baby. Our descriptions are illustrated by case histories and comments, some derived from hospital records but most extracted from a questionnaire survey of women who have suffered pre-eclampsia, carried out especially for this book. We begin with the mother's problems and how they can culminate in third-stage illness.

HIGH BLOOD PRESSURE

In pre-eclampsia the blood pressure is raised because of spasm in the small arteries, which increases their resistance to flow. The heart attempts to compensate for this problem and avert the threat of reduced blood flow to the organs and tissues by pumping harder, so that blood is forced through the constricted arteries at a higher pressure. Sometimes the heart does not compensate as fully as it should and the result is a sluggish flow running at a less raised or even, rarely, a normal pressure. In such cases pre-eclampsia can be very severe without very high blood pressure, so it is wrong to think of high blood pressure as a universal and essential sign of the disease.

No-one knows exactly what causes the small arteries to go into spasm in the first place, but there is increasing evidence that the process is triggered by damage to the endothelial cells, which make up the inner lining of all the body's blood vessels (see Chapter 6, p. 137).

The raised blood pressure of pre-eclampsia is not necessarily its most important feature, but it is emphasized by doctors and midwives for two reasons:

1. It is one of the earliest detectable signs of the condition, and so offers a useful warning of what may follow.
2. It is the easiest change to discern.

Many other changes are provoked by the sick placenta, but most can be detected only by elaborate and expensive tests, which are less acceptable to mothers and less practicable for the staff of busy antenatal clinics. Blood pressure measurement, on the other hand, is quick, cheap, painless and safe, so it is regarded as a convenient means of discovering and monitoring the progress of pre-eclampsia. From the medical point of view, the test offers a narrow but reasonably reliable window through which to 'see' the disease. We say 'reasonably' reliable because, although the severity of the hypertension usually reflects the severity of the underlying disease, this is not always true. And just as very severe pre-eclampsia—or even eclampsia—can be present without very high blood pressure, so it is possible to have very high blood pressure with relatively mild pre-eclampsia, as the two following case histories demonstrate.

Mild hypertension but severe pre-eclampsia

At exactly 33 weeks in her first pregnancy, Mrs A woke in the night with acute upper abdominal pain. She was admitted to hospital in the early hours and found to have a slightly raised blood pressure—130/90—and one 'plus' of protein in her urine. Blood samples were taken to check liver and clotting functions and, because the pain rapidly subsided and her blood pressure returned to normal, Mrs A was left to catch up on her sleep.

Over the next 2 days she felt well, with no pain and normal blood pressure, but with a persistent 'plus' of protein in her urine. Because her admission had coincided with a change in doctors' shifts, and because her symptoms had improved so rapidly, no-one had bothered to check the results of her blood tests until a relatively junior midwife came to file them in the notes.

She noted that Mrs A's platelet count on admission 3 days earlier was much lower than it should have been, and promptly called the obstetrician, who carried out another blood test. The low platelet count was not merely confirmed, it had fallen much further and was now so low that Mrs A was at risk of total breakdown of her clotting system. Her liver function tests were also found to be abnormal. Yet Mrs A still felt perfectly well, with a normal blood pressure, and the only other sign of her dangerous illness was the sinister 'plus' of protein.

After appropriate precautions to protect Mrs A from haemorrhage, her baby was delivered that same day by Caesarean section. Both mother and baby did well and 6 days later Mrs A's platelet count was totally normal.

Severe hypertension but mild pre-eclampsia

Mrs B, aged 25, got off to a good start in her first pregnancy, despite a history of chronic hypertension requiring permanent treatment. Her blood pressure, which registered 160/100 at 8 weeks, had fallen to 140/90 at 15 weeks, following the normal trend. However, by 23 weeks it had risen to

200/130, which looked ominously like severe early-onset pre-eclampsia, particularly as proteinuria had also set in.

However, Mrs B had no other signs of severe pre-eclampsia, with a normally grown baby, a normal blood concentration of uric acid and no evidence of disturbances of the clotting system. So her doctors decided to monitor her closely in hospital but to allow the pregnancy to continue.

Mrs B's blood pressure could never be adequately controlled and frequently reached 200/130, but her baby continued to grow and, apart from continuing proteinuria, no other signs of pre-eclampsia developed.

At 35 weeks Mrs B was induced—more because of medical nervousness about the level of her blood pressure than any deterioration in her condition —and delivered a healthy, normally-grown son. Six weeks later her blood pressure had settled to 148/98 and the proteinuria had disappeared.

In this latter case it must be presumed that Mrs B had some degree of pre-eclampsia, which seemed much more severe than it really was because of her underlying medical problem.

Pre-eclamptic hypertension may develop at any time in the second half of pregnancy, sometimes as late as during labour or even after delivery. The blood pressure is not just high but also unstable, so that it fluctuates wildly for no apparent reason.

Under normal circumstances, blood pressure is highest in the evening, falling dramatically overnight during sleep. But in pre-eclampsia the overnight drop in pressure does not usually happen, and sometimes the normal pattern is completely reversed, with the highest readings recorded during sleep or first thing in the morning. This unpredictability is hard to cope with, particularly for women being monitored in hospital, who can be reduced to despair by the lack of logic in what is going on; at moments of contented relaxation their blood pressure may be very high, while in stressful times it may be unaccountably low. 'What am I doing wrong', is the usual anxious question, to which the answer is always 'absolutely nothing'. The body is simply trying to keep pace with erratic signals coming from the placenta.

The confusion women feel in these circumstances arises from a largely mistaken view that people are responsible for their own blood pressures and can raise or lower them according to what they are doing or feeling. All too often women with pre-eclampsia blame themselves for their high blood pressure, seeing it as a direct result of anxiety or stress. Some women even fall prey to the dangerous delusion that if they could only escape from the unrestful environ-

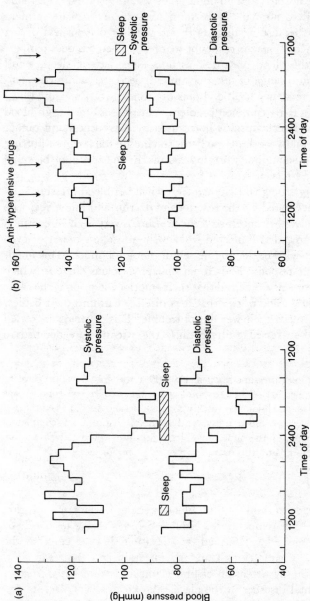

Fig. 4.1 Comparison of blood pressure recordings over 24 hours in normal and pre-eclamptic pregnancy. Chart (a) shows hour-by-hour fluctuations in blood pressure in a hospital patient with no blood pressure problems at 37 weeks of pregnancy; chart (b) shows fluctuations in a pre-eclamptic woman, also 37 weeks pregnant, being treated with antihypertensive drugs. The main difference, apart from the higher readings in the abnormal record, is the response to sleep: normally blood pressure falls during sleep, but in very severe pre-eclampsia it can sometimes show the opposite pattern, with the highest readings recorded during sleep.

ment of the hospital and go home, they would relax and their blood pressure fall to normal. 'Hypertension' is an unfortunate term in this respect because it suggests that tension or nervousness is part of the problem. There is no doubt that feeling nervous does temporarily raise the blood pressure—as does pain, lack of sleep, a full bladder, and a range of other stimuli. Indeed the 'white coat syndrome'—a tendency for blood pressure to rise when measured by a doctor—is a fairly common problem. But the sustained high blood pressure of pre-eclampsia is not caused by nervousness and cannot be brought on by working too hard, staying up too late, not putting your feet up enough or worrying too much; and it cannot be cured with rest and relaxation.

The worry a pregnant woman feels when her blood pressure is up is often exacerbated by the reactions of doctors and midwives, who may themselves be concerned if the pressure is very high. A common reaction is to tell the affected woman she must rest more, or even to chide her with neglecting herself or doing too much. This unfair and ignorant response leads to an unhappy vicious circle in which pregnant women, convinced that their emotional tension is the cause of their illness and, worse, that it is directly harming their babies, attempt to 'relax' their way out of trouble. This generates increased anxiety and increased guilt, because the attempts are doomed to failure.

When my blood pressure reached 150/100 I was told I would have to come in for bed rest—24–48 hours was suggested at the time. I was determined to get home as quickly as possible and so did everything I could to lower my blood pressure. I assumed that if I lay completely still and rested all the time, my blood pressure would fall to a more acceptable level. But this was not the case, and in fact it was up and down like a yo-yo.

Beverley Johnston

It is far better to think of high blood pressure in the same way you think of a high temperature. No-one believes that a fever can be caused by tension or banished by relaxation. It is accepted as the consequence of infection. Cure the infection and the fever goes. Similarly, the hypertension of pre-eclampsia is the consequence of a fundamental disorder in the placenta; take away the placenta and the blood pressure eventually falls.

In most cases of pre-eclampsia the blood pressure remains within limits that cause no overt problems. But occasionally it rises so high that the blood vessels are in danger of bursting. This is the point of transition between a symptomless second-stage sign and a dangerous third-stage illness, sometimes signalled by severe headache.

The most vulnerable vessels in the circulatory system are in the brain. If uncontrollably high pressure causes an artery to rupture here, then a *cerebral haemorrhage* (stroke) ensues. This is a well-known complication of severe hypertension in non-pregnant individuals and the most common cause of death in women with pre-eclampsia or eclampsia.

As far as is known, cerebral haemorrhage is the most significant (and very rare) consequence of extreme hypertension and it is to keep this complication at bay that antihypertensive drugs are prescribed in pre-eclampsia, although they cannot halt the progress of the underlying disease.

Before leaving the subject of high blood pressure, it is important to point out that the baby neither suffers high blood pressure itself nor is damaged by the mother's hypertension. The placental circulation on the mother's side is exposed to the raised pressure, but this does not appear to cause any of the problems that can affect a baby in pre-eclampsia.

SWELLING, FLUID RETENTION, AND WEIGHT GAIN

The one visible sign of second stage pre-eclampsia is swelling (oedema), but this is not a reliable sign for two reasons. First, oedema is also a common feature of normal, healthy pregnancy; indeed, there is good evidence that women who don't swell at all tend to produce smaller, slightly more vulnerable babies than those who do, although no-one knows why. Secondly, oedema is not a prerequisite for pre-eclampsia, and it is possible to have the full-blown disease without any swelling at all. Furthermore, this type of 'dry' pre-eclampsia, which accounts for about 1 in 4 of all cases, is known to be more dangerous than the 'wet' variety, although, again, it is not known why this should be.

Swelling in both normal and pre-eclamptic pregnancies is caused by retention of fluid—water, to be precise—in the tissues. This can be seen moving under the skin if a swollen area is pressed with a finger or thumb: the fluid in the area being compressed spreads into the surrounding tissues then, when the pressure is removed, an obvious dent remains for several seconds until the displaced fluid moves back.

Excess water accumulates most noticeably in the ankles and fingers but can be retained practically anywhere, including the face. Wherever it is retained it is inextricably bound up with weight gain —water is a very heavy substance. However, while the swelling of normal pregnancy tends to come on gradually, linked with a steady rate of weight gain, pre-eclamptic oedema is often sudden, severe and accompanied by an accelerated rate of weight gain.

The oedema was so severe that I appeared to have no neck, shoulders, knees or ankles. I resembled a Michelin man and actually 'sloshed' when I walked.

Anon.

What constitutes excessive weight gain in pregnancy? Unreasonably low limits have been set in the past: for example, Gordon Bourne in his respected handbook *Pregnancy* (Pan Books, 1984) lays down an overall limit of 8–9 kg (that is, 17–20 lb) for the whole pregnancy and argues that a weight gain of more than 10 lb between 20 and 30 weeks 'predisposes to pre-eclampsia'. However, it is probably fair to say that sudden swelling linked with a gain of more than 1 kg (2.2 lb) per week over 2 or 3 weeks should set off the warning bells. There are exceptions, as always, with pre-eclampsia, but this is a good general guideline, which justifies the inclusion of regular, accurate weighing in routine antenatal checks.

Why do pre-eclamptic women retain so much fluid

'Am I drinking too much?' some women ask, once again blaming themselves for events that are entirely outside their control. 'Definitely not', is the answer.

Control of the distribution of fluid is one of the body's most important functions as we are, after all, made up predominantly of water. Most of this water is held inside the cells—the basic building blocks of our tissues; some is in the blood, and the rest forms what is known as *interstitial fluid*, filling out the tiny spaces between the cells and blood vessels and providing a moist, spongy 'ground' for the cells to inhabit. The excess water of pre-eclampsia is retained in this interstitial fluid, from which it cannot be readily excreted. By contrast, the fluid volume of the blood tends to be reduced in pre-eclampsia, and this leads the kidneys to retain even more fluid, which ultimately aggravates the swelling.

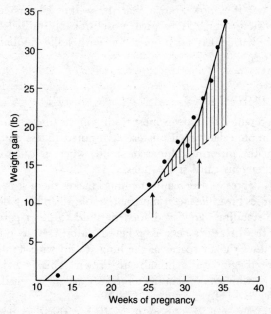

Fig. 4.2 Excessive weight gain in pre-eclampsia. The chart shows an abnormal pattern of weight gain in a patient who developed pre-eclampsia at 34 weeks. Her weight gain was normal until 26 weeks, when it suddenly accelerated (shown by the arrow) as she retained extra fluid, with another acceleration at around 32 weeks. The dashed line shows the expected rate of weight gain and the shaded area marks the excessive gain.

No-one knows exactly what causes the water retention and the associated blood volume reduction, but the best available explanation is that the blood vessels, particularly the body's vast network of tiny capillaries, are unduly 'leaky' in pre-eclampsia, allowing water to drain out of the bloodstream into the interstitial fluid, and thus waterlog the tissues.

It should be clearer now why drinking has nothing to do with fluid retention. Drinking too much or drinking less cannot affect the leakiness of the capillaries. They are leaky because they have been damaged in some way by the sick placenta.

Overeating

Overeating is also a red herring in pre-eclampsia. Doctors used to urge pregnant women who gained excessive weight to curb their appetites but it is now known that the weight gain is caused by fluid retention, which is in turn most probably caused by leaky capillaries. Eating has no more to do with leaky capillaries than drinking has.

'Hidden' oedema

Although retained fluid pools most readily in the limbs, extremities, and face, in pre-eclampsia it can also accumulate in less visible areas, such as in the intestines, lungs or brain, where it can sometimes lead to dangerous third-stage illness.

A small degree of oedema in the lungs makes them stiffer, which in turn causes breathlessness, most noticeable when lying down. On sitting or standing, gravity drains the fluid to other parts of the body so the breathlessness is relieved. More severe pulmonary oedema causes the air spaces of the lungs to fill with fluid, so that the sufferer begins quite literally to drown. This is a dangerous emergency, which may require temporary use of a ventilator (see Chapter 5, p. 116).

Oedema can cause the larynx to swell, but this does not usually cause problems unless a general anaesthetic is given, when the anaesthetist finds it difficult or even impossible to introduce an airway into the windpipe. Oedema in the abdominal cavity causes swelling but no problems. The retained fluid is discovered and released at Caesarean section and can easily amount to 3 or 4 pints. Oedema in the brain is more serious as it can lead to fits (see p. 80).

THE KIDNEYS AND PROTEIN IN THE URINE

The appearance of an abnormal amount of protein in the urine—a sign that kidney function is beginning to deteriorate—is one of the most important landmarks in the development of pre-eclampsia. It marks the transition from an early, relatively benign, phase of second-stage disease (non-proteinuric pre-eclampsia) to an advanced, unstable phase (proteinuric pre-eclampsia).

The expected 'life' of a pregnancy from the time that protein becomes persistently present in the urine is about 14 days. Unless the baby has been delivered by then, the mother is likely to develop serious, even life-threatening third-stage illness. However, 14 days is merely an average and for some women it may be as little as a day or two, while for others it may be as much as a month—even 6 weeks. The trouble is that there is no way of predicting when disaster will strike in any particular case, which is why it is essential for women with proteinuric pre-eclampsia to be monitored in hospital.

The problem from the mother's point of view is that she still feels very well and it is almost impossible for her to believe that danger is so imminent. Of course in her case it may *not* be, although as a rule the longer the proteinuria persists the nearer to danger she comes, not because the proteinuria is dangerous or harmful in itself, but because the disease is naturally progressive and time always makes it worse.

Measuring protein in the urine

The dipstick test, which enables doctors to detect protein in the urine, is only a rough screening process and can give false results from time to time. The results are usually recorded as 'trace' (of protein), '+', '++' and so on up to four 'plusses'. The 'trace' result often means nothing and can be ignored. But '+' or more must be taken seriously: if the reading is correct it means that there is definitely more protein in the urine than there should be, although it is impossible to say how much more because the test measures the *concentration* of protein in the urine, not the *total amount*. If a woman is dehydrated, her urine will be more concentrated than usual and the apparent protein content exaggerated. If, on the other hand, she is drinking a lot, the urine will be very dilute and the protein content underestimated. So a positive result should be checked, if there is time, by a 24-hour urine collection, in which the total amount of protein lost over a complete day and night can be measured. This gives a true indication of how much protein is in the urine—and in' general the greater the proteinuria the worse the disease.

Where does the protein come from?

How does it relate to what most people, particularly pregnant women, think of as an essential part of their diet?

Proteins are among the basic substances of life. Indeed, the sole function of our genes, which contain our complete inheritance from our parents, is to control the production of proteins by each and every one of the body's cells. So proteins are everywhere within us. Naturally, some are in the blood, where they carry messages or nourishment or have other useful functions to perform. Because these proteins are useful to the body, the filters in the kidneys are designed to retain them in the bloodstream, not to waste them in the urine. But in pre-eclampsia the filters are damaged, as a result of the changes in the sick placenta. This makes them 'leaky', so that the protein normally retained in the blood is lost in the urine. No-one knows what causes this leakiness in the kidney's filtering units (the glomeruli), but the evidence suggests that the problem, like the arterial spasm that raises the blood pressure, is caused by damage to the endothelial cells lining all the body's blood vessels.

Each glomerulus (there are at least a million of these microscopic structures in each kidney) is made up of a small knot of capillaries suspended in a tiny cup. Plasma, the fluid portion of the blood, is pushed out of the capillaries into the cup, from where it trickles away down a long thin tubule to be turned into urine. The endothelial cells lining the glomerular capillaries form the first layer of the filter. In pre-eclampsia they become swollen, bulging out into, and blocking, the hollow part of the capillaries. It is easy to see how this might damage the filtering function of the glomeruli, so that proteins that should remain in the bloodstream leak out into the fluid that becomes urine.

However, this is not the full extent of the damage. Because blood flow through all affected glomeruli is likely to be reduced, waste products such as urea and creatinine are excreted less efficiently than usual and tend to accumulate in the bloodstream, where their concentration rises. So abnormally high concentrations of creatinine and urea in the blood may also be a sign of second-stage pre-eclampsia. But, like protein in the urine, these are signs of advanced involvement of the kidneys. Other kidney functions are impaired before this, particularly the ability to excrete another waste product —uric acid. So abnormally high blood levels of uric acid can be an earlier sign of pre-eclampsia.

The accumulation of these waste products in the bloodstream poses no direct dangers to mother or baby as long as the kidneys continue working. Unfortunately, in rare cases impaired function gives rise to total kidney failure, a dangerous third-stage complication from which most women make a complete recovery, although it is possible to suffer irretrievable damage.

Irreversible kidney failure

Mrs C had enjoyed a perfectly healthy first pregnancy—indeed she had been so confident that everything was absolutely normal that she had booked for a home delivery. But at 32 weeks she developed ankle oedema and slightly raised blood pressure, which grew steadily worse until she was finally admitted to hospital with severe pre-eclampsia 3 weeks later.

Mrs C was treated with bed rest and antihypertensives, but her blood pressure became more and more difficult to control. Nevertheless, when she was delivered by emergency Caesarean a week after admission, it was less for her own sake than for her baby, who was showing signs of distress.

After the delivery Mrs C was expected to make a rapid recovery, but that night two dramatic complications arose: her blood pressure shot up and could not be brought down and her urine flow first slowed and finally stopped, indicating total kidney failure.

After 3 days in a coma, Mrs C began to recover with the aid of an artificial kidney machine. She was assured that her own kidneys would soon take over again—as they do in 99 per cent of similar pre-eclamptic crises—but in fact she never regained any useful kidney function.

A kidney transplant carried out 9 months later was unsuccessful, and for the past 10 years Mrs C has relied on dialysis to compensate for her failed kidneys. She describes her quality of life as 'virtually normal' and continues to work part time. But her life expectation, even with dialysis, is uncertain.

High blood pressure, swelling, and protein in the urine are all most women know of pre-eclampsia; but the disease can have much farther reaching effects, causing disturbances to the liver, the nervous system, and the blood clotting system. Indeed, it is possible that no function of the body is exempt from the potential repercussions of this strange condition.

CLOTTING PROBLEMS

Enhanced 'clottability' of the blood is a normal feature of pregnancy, facilitated by an increased concentration of several circulating clotting factors and greater reactivity of the platelets, the specialized blood cells responsible for clotting.

Pre-eclampsia sometimes makes the platelets even *more* reactive, so they are used up at a faster rate than normal and their concentration in blood is consequently reduced. Other circulating components of the clotting system may also show small changes.

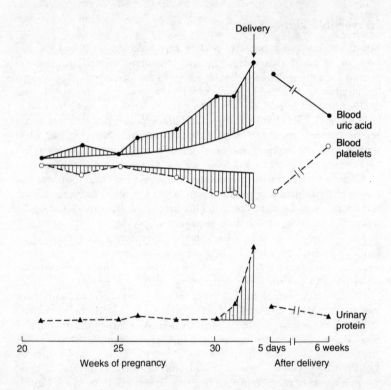

Fig. 4.3 Platelets, protein, and uric acid in pre-eclampsia. The chart shows changes in blood levels of platelets and uric acid and the concentration of protein in the urine of a patient who developed severe pre-eclampsia at 30 weeks and had to be delivered at 32 weeks. The lowest line shows the onset of proteinuria, typically at two weeks before delivery. The two upper lines show a much earlier—and simultaneous—reduction in platelets and increase in plasma uric acid. In each case the shaded areas mark departures from the norm.

The concentration of platelets in a blood sample can be measured quickly and accurately. During normal pregnancy the numbers vary from individual to individual, over a range of 150 000–350 000 per cubic millimetre of blood. A persistent fall in the count or a sudden dramatic reduction can be detected in some cases even before proteinuria appears. In other cases the functioning of the platelets is disturbed but their concentration in the blood remains unaffected. These second-stage changes do not throw the clotting system off balance and it continues to do its job more or less as it should. However, in rare cases, the disturbances are so extreme that the clotting system destabilizes and goes out of control, leading to purposeless and highly dangerous clotting in small blood vessels all over the body—a third-stage complication known as *disseminated intravascular coagulation* (DIC). So many small blood vessels become blocked by these inappropriate clots that the circulation to vital organs like the heart, liver, kidneys, and brain begins to fail; but there is an even more dangerous consequence—haemorrhage.

As widespread, uncontrollable clotting in the small blood vessels uses up all the fuel for clotting throughout the body, the liquid blood that remains to maintain the circulation is stripped clean of its clotting factors, so it simply cannot clot. This means that even the tiniest pinprick injury to a blood vessel becomes a permanent leak, oozing blood for many hours.

Under such circumstances delivery or other surgery is extremely hazardous, as the mother could well bleed to death.

Another aspect of this horrific complication is that the body's red blood cells become severely damaged in attempting to force their way through abnormal clots in all the capillaries. As a result they tend to burst and release their contents—a process known as *haemolysis*.

LIVER DAMAGE

The potential for liver damage in pre-eclampsia is often not sufficiently emphasized. It tends to be a fairly late feature of the disease and is hard to detect, except through blood tests, which can reveal leakage of the contents of damaged liver cells into the bloodstream.

The causes of this liver damage are not known but the most likely explanation is that the sick placenta causes general damage to the circulation, thus provoking abnormal clotting and depriving the liver, as well as other essential organs, of their full blood supply. Liver damage is usually linked with involvement of the clotting system and, in extreme cases, a combined breakdown of the liver and clotting system can ensue (see below).

Jaundice, a common sign of liver problems, does not usually occur with pre-eclampsia but there are, as always, exceptions and some women turn yellow as the disease progresses. As the pre-eclampsia evolves the damaged liver swells, stretching its protective capsule. This capsule is very sensitive and the stretching causes pain, which is sometimes aggravated by bleeding under the capsule. This stretching and bleeding is the cause of the abdominal pain felt just under the ribs by some women with advanced pre-eclampsia—a symptom often mistakenly ascribed to heartburn or even gallstones. In very rare cases the liver swells so much that it bursts. This is, not surprisingly, a major third-stage calamity, requiring emergency surgery to save the mother's life.

The HELLP syndrome

Another perilous third-stage complication is a combined breakdown of the liver and clotting system known as the *HELLP syndrome* —*H*aemolysis (see p. 73), *E*levated *L*iver enzymes (liver enzymes accumulate in the blood as the liver cells leak their contents), *L*ow *P*latelets (see p. 72). Sometimes this complication is seen without the haemolysis, when it may be called the *ELLP syndrome*.

When I finished my full-time employment as a secretary at 30 weeks I felt fit and healthy and was receiving plenty of comments on how marvellous I looked. But at 31 weeks I became ill literally overnight. I started getting contractions every 10 minutes and passing urine constantly. I also developed a never-ending thirst. These were the first signs of pregnancy-induced diabetes, but were originally treated as a urine infection. A few days later I was found to have high blood pressure and protein in my urine and developed a persistent indigestion-type pain.

I was in hospital less than a week before they had to deliver my baby. My blood pressure remained high and the protein in my urine increased. I had this indigestion pain all the time, but it wasn't until they realized I had liver problems that the source of the pain was recognized.

My blood was being constantly tested because of the diabetes and one day, during one of these tests, my blood spurted out over the bedclothes. An hour or so later during a finger prick test my blood spurted all over the nurse's uniform. A blood specialist from a neighbouring hospital was called to see me, and it was then realized that the platelets in my blood had failed, preventing my blood from clotting properly, and also that my liver had started to fail.

When they decided to do a Caesarean section they told my parents that they would know in 24 hours whether I was going to survive. Before surgery I had eight bags of clotting agent run through a drip and a number of injections to build up the baby's lungs in preparation for early delivery. Kevin was born at 33 weeks, weighing 5 lb 2 oz, and was able to breathe without a ventilator.

I spent the next 2 days in intensive care. I could not move as at one point I was attached to eight drips and a catheter. I was lifted out of bed for the first time on the fifth day: I had lost all the weight from the pregnancy plus half a stone, so I weighed 6½ stone. I had a very low blood count and my wound had developed an infection. While I was recovering in hospital I felt like a celebrity. Practically every doctor and midwife in the hospital came to see me. I was told I had suffered a very rare form of toxaemia called the HELLP syndrome, and the midwives told me they all had to read up on my case.

I left hospital two weeks after delivery but was not fully discharged until a few weeks later, when my liver and platelets had returned to normal and the diabetes had cleared up. It took me at least 6 months after delivery to return to normal health. I had a low blood count for months and did not regain my normal weight for a year.

After my experiences I can't see myself having any more children, but when I look at Kevin, now a year old, it all seems worthwhile.

Anna Brown

THE THIRD STAGE OF PRE-ECLAMPSIA

This is when serious illness begins to develop and, for the first time, the mother feels unwell. Her symptoms are a sign that her body's systems are breaking down, beginning to go out of control and losing their normal precisely-regulated balance.

Typical symptoms of third-stage pre-eclampsia are:

Headache

The headache accompanying the third-stage of pre-eclampsia is often described as 'the worst headache in my life'. The pain may be at the front, top or back of the head or simply 'all over'. Sometimes the pain is felt at the back of the neck, extending upwards, and is described as 'neckache' rather than headache.

It was fortunate that I had been admitted to hospital as one afternoon, quite suddenly, my slight headache became the most dreadful one, accompanied by flashing lights. I felt so awful that I couldn't even summon the strength to call for a nurse. At that time they were checking my blood pressure each hour and when the next check came round I managed to say how bad I felt. I have never seen people move so quickly. My bed was taken at top speed into a darkened quiet room and I was given an injection. The following day I felt better and my daughter's birth was induced.

Maureen Clark

Visual disturbances

The headache may be associated with disturbances in vision such as flashing or multicoloured lights, which are similar to the 'aura' preceding migraine attacks.

Six weeks prior to my due date I was at an antenatal clinic when I developed 'migrainous' symptoms—flashing lights, numbness, inability to speak coherently, etc. I suffer badly with migraine and thought little of it, although I did mention it to the doctors. My blood pressure was found to be high and I was admitted to hospital . . .

Polly Vincent

This symptom can cause confusion because many migraine sufferers continue with their attacks during pregnancy and others may experience migraine for the first time.

In rare cases, pre-eclampsia can actually damage the vision, leading to temporary or even permanent blindness. The retina of the eye—the thin membrane where light and colours are detected and converted into signals interpreted by the brain—can become detached from the eyeball, probably as a result of oedema within the eye. With appropriate treatment, the retina can reattach itself and full recovery of sight is possible.

Another rare problem is 'cortical blindness', in which the part of the brain that interprets the retinal signals is damaged by the circulatory problems of pre-eclampsia. So, although the eyes work perfectly well, the brain is unable to make sense of what they see. Most people recover their sight eventually, but there are exceptions.

Abdominal pain/vomiting

A common symptom of very severe pre-eclampsia is pain in the abdomen, especially in the upper part under the ribs, either in the middle or to the right, which comes from stretching of the liver capsule (see p. 73). This type of pain, often accompanied by nausea and/or vomiting is frequently misdiagnosed or overlooked.

At 32½ weeks I had terrible pains in my chest around the breast bone and back, and I couldn't sleep. I used Raljex (a pain-relieving preparation applied to the skin) but eventually this was no help. Everyone presumed this was just a normal discomfort of pregnancy. I went to see my GP, but he found nothing discernible, although I forgot to take a urine sample with me on this occasion. The GP prescribed sleeping tablets and embrocation—the sort used by athletes—to put on the painful areas. He didn't mention that the symptoms could be due to toxaemia.

The pain and sleeplessness got worse and I could only get relief by lying directly in front of the gas fire. I continued with my embrocation and sleeping tablets until I went for my hospital antenatal appointment at 34½ weeks. On this occasion my blood pressure was 170/100 and I had four 'plusses' of protein in my urine.

I was admitted for bed rest, but as soon as I was examined by a doctor it was decided that I needed to be delivered immediately by Caesarean section . . . I certainly didn't realize how serious toxaemia could be or I wouldn't have gone to the doctor without a sample or waited so long between hospital visits. As it was, the symptoms were overlooked until a very late stage.

Susan Turner

The most dramatic of all third-stage symptoms is a convulsive seizure, which marks the transition from pre-eclampsia to eclampsia.

ECLAMPSIA—THE ONSET OF CONVULSIONS

Pre-eclampsia is so named because it was originally identified as a disorder preceding eclampsia, although it is now known that eclamptic convulsions are only one of several potential complications of the disease.

These convulsions, which lead to temporary loss of consciousness, look no different from epileptic fits. The mother is gripped by synchronized, repetitive, jerky, and sometimes quite violent movements involving muscle groups in the eyes, jaw, neck, and limbs. The spasms stop the mother from breathing, make her bite her tongue and sometimes cause urinary incontinence. Most convulsions last for a minute or less before stopping spontaneously. If they are continuous, without a break, the woman is said to be in *status eclampticus* and is in extreme danger—initially from suffocation, then from brain damage.

Eclamptic fits are triggered by abnormal activity in the nerve cells of the brain; when these cells are damaged, as they can be by the pre-eclamptic process, their highly-organized activity can become so disturbed that it explodes into intense electrical discharges, which stimulate the convulsive movements.

Eclamptic fits usually occur as a third-stage complication of severe pre-eclampsia. But sometimes they arise out of the blue, without any evidence of preceding disturbances, although in these cases other signs of pre-eclampsia tend to appear at the same time as the fits.

Eclampsia can occur at any time in the second half of pregnancy —or even earlier in rare cases. In 1974, a case of eclampsia at 16 weeks was reported in the *Journal of the American Medical Association*. At the other extreme, the fits can occur as late as during labour or after delivery; in fact one case has been reported as late as 3 weeks after delivery.

A late case of eclampsia

Mrs D's first pregnancy ended with a miscarriage. She had inherited a tendency to chronic hypertension from her mother, and early in her second pregnancy her blood pressure was above average at 140–160/80–90. Nevertheless, the pregnancy progressed well until 38 weeks, when her diastolic pressure rose first to 110 and then to 120 and protein started to appear in her urine. She was admitted to hospital and treated with methyldopa (an antihypertensive drug).

Mrs D was induced at 39 weeks, given an epidural anaesthetic to help control her blood pressure, which did not rise above 145/100 during labour, and delivered a healthy, well-grown daughter. On the fifth day after delivery she was discharged at her own insistence, although she had persisting proteinuria and was still taking tablets for her blood pressure.

Two days later, after suffering increasingly severe headaches, she had two major eclamptic convulsions at home and was readmitted and treated with Valium and phenytoin (an anticonvulsant drug) to prevent further fits. Her blood pressure now rose as high as 200/115 and the antihypertensive treatment had to be stepped up considerably to control it. Six weeks later she was off all medication and her blood pressure had settled to normal.

It is unusual for a woman to feel totally well before an eclamptic fit. She may become restless and 'shaky'; or she may suffer intense headache or visual disturbances. However, if there have been no preceding signs of pre-eclampsia, the fits tend to occur without warning symptoms, typically during labour or immediately afterwards. Eclampsia of this kind is usually much milder than when it complicates severe pre-eclampsia because all the mother's problems seem to be localized in her brain and there are few, if any, other disturbances. So although the symptoms are very dramatic, they do not reflect a particularly profound illness and recovery is generally rapid.

My blood pressure remained at 110/60 or 120/70 throughout my pregnancy and at no stage did I have protein in my urine. My total weight gain was 2 stones, which wasn't considered excessive. The first sign of trouble was when I was admitted to hospital in the early stages of labour at 40 weeks, when my blood pressure registered 150/110. However, it went down as labour progressed and only increased again as I reached 10 cm dilation, at which point I suffered the first of two eclamptic fits.

I remember nothing about these fits or the emergency Caesarean delivery that followed. When I was told, I was utterly shocked: I had had a model pregnancy—no morning sickness even!—and am generally healthy, athletic, and vigorous. I am told that I recovered well after delivery, although I was anaemic and had to stay in hospital for 12 days.

Emma Padmore

As convulsions cause loss of consciousness, women with eclampsia cannot normally remember this part of their illness, and their amnesia is compounded by the sedative drugs that are given to control the fits. The baby often has to be delivered urgently, by Caesarean section, under general anaesthetic, which makes the whole episode even more confused, chaotic and unpleasant.

At 36 weeks I was admitted with high blood pressure, oedema and protein in the urine. That same day I remember having a headache and the doctors telling me that I would have to have a Caesarean as my blood pressure was so high. I remember being prepared for the Caesarean and then nothing else until 3 days later.

I was in intensive care for 2 days, in a coma, on a life-support machine. When I came round I wasn't even aware that I had been in intensive care, and when I was told what had happened by a member of my family I felt petrified that I had come so close to death. My first feeling was gratitude that I was alive. Later on I felt anger and confusion that my pregnancy had ended this way. Physically I recovered very quickly, but mentally it took about a year.

Bonita Pearcey

There is no one cause of eclampsia and several factors are probably involved in its genesis. These include:

1. *Swelling in the brain* (cerebral oedema), possibly as a complication of excessive fluid retention.
2. *Reduced blood flow to the brain* caused by a combination of small clots and spasm of the small arteries.
3. *Bleeding from small arteries* ruptured by the intensity of the blood pressure.

Any eclamptic woman is at risk of suffocation while the seizure is happening. But a woman who passes this hurdle may still be at risk depending on the degree of brain damage that triggered the fit in the first place. While swelling in the brain is easily reversed, a brain haemorrhage is not. Whereas minor spasm of the arteries is usually a temporary problem, severe constriction, leading to the death of nerve cells in part of the brain, causes permanent damage.

Most women make a full recovery from eclampsia. But some are left with permanent disability, while a tragic few are so badly brain-damaged that their existence is little short of vegetative.

MATERNAL DEATH

Pregnancies that end in death, either of mother or baby, are among the great tragedies of life; what should be a joyful and creative event is not merely frustrated but perverted in the most awful of ways. There are few people who can cope with the idea of this happening, let alone the reality.

Thankfully it is very, very rare these days for pregnant women to die of pre-eclampsia or eclampsia. This is partly because of improved general health and partly because doctors and midwives have been increasingly successful in limiting the damage caused by the disease. Nevertheless, pre-eclampsia and eclampsia are still the most common causes of maternal deaths in the Western world, killing about 10 women every year in the UK. These numbers are so insignificant in comparison to deaths from cancer, heart disease, suicide, road accidents, and AIDS that the disease has never been considered a very important public health issue. Nevertheless, most people find it immensely shocking to think of any woman dying in these circumstances.

Most victims die of brain damage, particularly strokes resulting from cerebral haemorrhage. Intractable bleeding as a consequence of clotting disturbances is less commonly fatal, but still causes occasional deaths, and it is not unknown for a woman to die despite receiving more than 100 pints of transfused blood. Respiratory failure, heart failure, and liver failure are all potentially fatal complications, although kidney failure is treatable by dialysis.

It is a common misconception that pre-eclampsia is dangerous only when it culminates in convulsions. In fact, pre-eclampsia causes as many deaths as eclampsia itself.

As we pointed out in Chapter 1 (see p. 7), the *Reports on Confidential Enquiries into Maternal Deaths in England and Wales* have linked most maternal deaths to substandard care by doctors and/or midwives, and in theory it should be possible to abolish all such deaths by improving the quality of maternity services. It is difficult to assess how many more women would perish without the safety net of antenatal care, but we would probably be talking about hundreds rather than handfuls of deaths each year.

HOW LONG DOES THE ILLNESS LAST?

Pre-eclampsia, as we have said already, is an immensely variable and unpredictable condition, which obeys no rules and rarely follows a set pattern. For example, it usually becomes apparent at any time after 20 weeks, but cases of eclampsia have been known to occur even earlier and, although the disease should be well on the wane within a day or two of delivery, women have died of eclampsia as late as 5 days afterwards. Women who have been hospitalized antenatally often chafe at being kept in hospital after delivery: but how many of them are aware of the dangers they may still encounter?

Just as the time of onset varies, so does the speed with which the disease progresses. It may grumble on over several months or develop and build to a crisis in the space of a few days: such sudden, severe, and rapidly progressive disease is often described as *'fulminating pre-eclampsia'*.

The progress of the disorder is halted by delivery, so *when* a woman begins to get pre-eclampsia determines to a large extent how *severe* her case will be. Pre-eclampsia beginning at around full term is normally a trivial complication, and most cases fall into this category. But if the disease begins in the second trimester there will be plenty of time for it to build up to a dangerous illness, however slowly it does so.

Not everyone agrees on the distinction between mild and severe pre-eclampsia, but we would argue that while high blood pressure alone, with or without oedema, includes cases that can be classified as 'mild' pre-eclampsia, the appearance of abnormal amounts of protein in the urine marks a shift into severe disease, which is why all proteinuric patients should be kept in hospital until delivery.

One fairly consistent feature of pre-eclampsia is that once established it *always* gets worse until the baby is delivered; and it gets worse at a progressively faster rate!

Two main challenges face the doctors and midwives responsible for providing antenatal care. First, they must not miss any of the various signs of pre-eclampsia, which justifies the need for all those routine checks that so many women find so tedious. Secondly, once pre-eclampsia is diagnosed, they have to keep one step ahead of the disease so they are not caught out by any unexpected developments and so that they have time to deliver the baby before things become really serious.

WHAT HAPPENS TO THE BABY?

The baby's experience of pre-eclampsia is quite different from that of its mother. He or she has one major problem: how to survive with a damaged lifeline and a consequent shortage of oxygen and food.

Initially the baby adapts to oxygen shortage by enhancing the oxygen-carrying capacity of its blood. It does this by manufacturing more red blood cells, each loaded with the vital oxygen-carrying pigment, haemoglobin. As a result the baby becomes *polycythaemic*, which simply means that its blood is thicker than usual because of all the extra red cells. However, as the oxygen supply from the placenta is reduced still further, more critical internal adjustments have to be made and the baby's body begins to restrict the flow of blood to its limbs, guts, and kidneys to preserve the vital supply to the heart and brain. Finally there comes a point when the baby has no further reserves of oxygen to call on and its systems are in danger of breaking down. The baby has one desperate, last ditch measure up its sleeve: it can extract energy from its fuel supplies without oxygen. But this highly inefficient process generates a potentially poisonous waste product—lactic acid—and once this begins to accumulate the baby will die if not rescued by delivery.

Mothers can often tell when this crisis point has been reached because once a baby has flooded its body with lactic acid—a state known as *acidosis*—it becomes effectively unconscious and stops moving.

Doctors can also detect the onset of acidosis by monitoring the baby's heart rate electronically: the trace will be flatter than usual, with little variability of the interval between beats and unhealthy 'decelerations', a sign of acute oxygen starvation. It is routine practice for doctors to monitor the heart rates of babies affected by pre-eclampsia to pick up the earliest signs of suffocation (see Chapter 5, p. 104).

An oxygen-starved baby will be limp and unresponsive after delivery, and its blood will be unusually acidic and dark because of the low concentration of oxygen. However, babies are much tougher than we imagine and most make a complete recovery, even from such severe problems, although others sustain permanent damage.

The other consequence of reduced blood flow to the placenta is shortage of food for the baby. This progressive starvation has predictable results: the baby gets leaner and grows more slowly; and growth of vital organs like the brain is sustained at the expense of less vital structures such as the liver and other abdominal organs. Eventually all growth is bound to cease and, if the baby survives long enough to be delivered, it may be born suffering from an extreme form of malnutrition associated with famine-wracked Third World countries.

Starvation makes newborn babies particularly vulnerable because they have no food reserves to call on: no stores of fuel in the form of fat or carbohydrate. Glucose, the body's main fuel, is delivered to the baby via the umbilical cord throughout pregnancy, but the supply is suddenly severed at delivery. A healthy, well-nourished newborn can quickly mobilize alternative supplies from its stores, so that it needs no food apart from that provided by colostrum, the forerunner of breast milk until breast-feeding becomes established 2 or 3 days later. But the starved, growth-retarded baby has no way of sustaining the level of glucose in its blood after delivery because it has no stores, and unless supplementary glucose is given at once there is a serious risk of brain damage.

Fortunately, an adequate supply of food can normally be re-established after delivery, although this is not always easy if the baby is very premature. Many babies who have starved in the womb recover rapidly and catch up on their growth within a few months. But others have lost so much ground before delivery that they remain consistently small for their age.

I was admitted to hospital with fulminating pre-eclampsia—blood pressure 180/120, grotesque oedema and a lot of protein in my urine—at 29 weeks; Luke was delivered by emergency Caesarean section 2 days later.

Luke weighed 1.1 kg (2.4 lb) at birth. He had severe respiratory distress syndrome and required respiratory assistance for 4½ weeks. He developed a pneumothorax (air in the pleural cavity) and needed a chest drain. He also needed three top-up blood transfusions for anaemia.

Luke's progress was very slow and he experienced many setbacks. He was discharged home at 12 weeks, weighing less than 4 lb. Now aged 2¾ he appears 'normal' but has been very behind in reaching his milestones and has remained very small and prone to chest infections.

Jeannette Cooper

Some mothers believe their unborn babies' nutritional problems are somehow caused by their *own* eating habits and feel they should be able to improve matters by eating more or better. But in a normally well-nourished woman, such gross problems are caused by the failing placenta, not the mother's diet. The mother is sending ample supplies of oxygen and nourishment to the placenta, but the placenta is failing to pass them on to the baby.

The baby's growth inside the uterus can be monitored accurately by ultrasound measurements, usually of the girth of the abdomen. As the baby becomes progressively starved of food, the rate of growth first slows, then stops and, in the most extreme cases, may even go into reverse.

Baby deaths associated with pre-eclampsia are many times more common than maternal deaths. It is impossible to say for certain how many die each year, but in the UK it could amount to as many as 1000. Most of these babies die of the effects of premature delivery, which was necessary either to save their mothers' lives or to improve their own chances of survival.

I was in hospital for about 1½ weeks before my twin sons were delivered at 26 weeks. I woke in the night with backache, feeling very strange. My blood pressure was very high and I was given pills and monitored. A Caesarean was performed the following evening because of fear that I would suffer fits. One of the doctors told my husband that another 24 hours delay would make no difference to the babies but could make me a lot worse.

At the time I was excited to think my babies were going to be born— I didn't think at all about the consequences of them being born so early. The second twin Sam, who weighed only 652 g (1.4 lb), died after 5 days, but Mark, who weighed 1398 g (3 lb), battled on for 12½ weeks before he finally died. He had four operations, several bouts of jaundice and was very ill. He suffered a brain haemorrhage after about 4 days and, had he lived, would have been affected mentally and physically.

Sara Bestley

Some babies die as more mature stillbirths. In the days before high-tech monitoring was available this kind of death used to be quite common because it was impossible for doctors to assess which babies were in distress and in need of early delivery to save their lives. Nowadays, however, stillbirths tend to occur only when the disease has gone undetected or if the sick placenta separates prematurely from its anchorage in the uterus. This catastrophic event, known as *placental abruption*, usually kills the baby very quickly and may cause severe bleeding and other problems in the mother.

Fortunately, most babies survive pre-eclampsia and, if they are not too premature or malnourished, have an excellent outlook. The disease itself does not appear to carry any long-term risks beyond the knock-on consequences of suffocation, malnutrition or prematurity. Suffocation, if extreme, may cause permanent brain damage, such as cerebral palsy, and malnutrition may be so severe that the child never catches up on growth, although mental agility seems to be remarkably unaffected. A combination of extreme prematurity, malnutrition, and some degree of suffocation is highly likely to lead to some form of impairment, although this is not always severe.

HOW PRE-ECLAMPSIA IS DIAGNOSED

Given the dangers of pre-eclampsia and the speed at which it can progress, early diagnosis is vital to successful treatment. But diagnosis is fraught with problems of its own. For one thing, none of the clinical signs commonly associated with pre-eclampsia is completely specific to the disease—they can all have other causes. This means the diagnosis can be made only if at least two of the typical features are present, most commonly raised blood pressure and protein in the urine.

Raised blood pressure

Raised blood pressure is usually the first sign to become apparent at routine antenatal checks, but it can be confused with essential hypertension, although essential hypertension tends to reveal itself early in pregnancy and is not associated with other disturbances.

Proteinuria

Proteinuria is normally a later sign than hypertension, but doctors can seek earlier evidence of kidney involvement by measuring blood concentrations of the waste product uric acid, which are typically raised in pre-eclampsia.

Oedema

Oedema on its own is not a very useful sign because it is such a common feature of normal pregnancy. However, if the swelling comes on suddenly and is accompanied by rapid weight gain, amounting to more than 1 kg (2.2 lb) per week, it is more likely to be a sign of pre-eclampsia.

Blood clotting and liver function

Changes in blood clotting or liver function can be detected in blood tests. But these are signs of such advanced disease that the tests are more often used to monitor the extent of the problem than to diagnose it in the first place.

Reduced fetal growth

Another obvious sign to look for to confirm a possible diagnosis of pre-eclampsia is reduced fetal growth, although it is true that some babies continue to thrive even when their mothers are seriously ill.

Unfortunately, even with all these signs to look for, the diagnosis of pre-eclampsia is far from straightforward. One symptom alone is not enough to make a diagnosis and the absence of any one symptom is not enough to disprove it. Moreover, the condition can be so fast-moving that normality today cannot guarantee normality tomorrow. The main problem is that when the diagnosis is in doubt —as is often the case—there is no specific test to decide the issue one way or the other. This leads to endless arguments between doctors: some insist that pre-eclampsia can only be diagnosed in the presence of such and such a sign, or signs; others prefer a broader framework for the diagnosis. And at the moment there is no way of proving who is right.

Doctors' current problems with pre-eclampsia are similar to those they used to face in diagnosing tuberculosis (TB). Before the organism that causes TB was identified, diagnosis was a hit-and-miss affair, resting on the detection of such non-specific signs as fever, cough, and loss of weight. As each of these signs had other potential causes there was plenty of scope for disagreement and no proof one way or the other. Now, however, there is no room for dispute or error and TB can be diagnosed with absolute certainty by detecting the organism that causes it in samples of sputum. No-one can have TB without harbouring the organism, and its presence is indisputable evidence of the disease because it is the *prime cause*. Doctors still do not know the prime cause of pre-eclampsia and, until they do, there can be no specific test to establish the diagnosis beyond doubt.

The uncertainties of diagnosis are compounded by the elusive nature of the disease itself; it is a chameleon, which refuses to be stereotyped by diagnostic rules and whenever specialists, however experienced, think they have seen it all, along comes a new variant to take them by surprise.

Chronic or pre-eclamptic hypertension?

The most common difficulty, as we have already mentioned, is how to distinguish between pre-eclamptic and chronic hypertension. The distinction may seem academic, but it is important because chronic hypertension, however severe, has no direct ill effects on the outcome of the pregnancy. So women with non-pre-eclamptic hypertension do not need to be hospitalized, induced early or exposed to any of the treatments routinely given to women suffering from pre-eclampsia. However, these women do need to be monitored with extra vigilance in pregnancy because they are more at risk of pre-eclampsia—known in such cases as superimposed pre-eclampsia—than women with no pre-existing blood pressure problems.

The effects of chronic kidney disease

Chronic kidney disease can also increase a woman's risk of developing pre-eclampsia, although in such cases the disease can be extremely difficult to diagnose because kidney disease can also cause proteinuria and high blood pressure. It is not easy for doctors to distinguish between a worsening chronic problem and the onset of pre-eclampsia.

Pre-eclampsia can be so mild as to be barely discernible, or severe enough to threaten the mother's life. The first sign is normally high blood pressure, although it can be something unusual like jaundice; sometimes the mother is fine but poor growth in the baby rings warning bells; sometimes eclampsia occurs out of the blue with no preceding signs of pre-eclampsia. All these exceptions increase the difficulties of diagnosis. To detect the disease in all its guises requires vigilance, backed up by a lot of tedious monitoring. It also requires midwives and doctors who can recognize the early signs, and co-operation from the mothers themselves, a subject dealt with in Chapter 5.

WHO IS AT RISK?

First-time mothers are several times more prone to pre-eclampsia than those in second or subsequent pregnancies. Unfortunately, however, it is not true that after suffering pre-eclampsia in a first pregnancy you will not get it again.

In fact, the women most likely to suffer pre-eclampsia in a second pregnancy are those who have had it before, while those who enjoy a normal first pregnancy have an extremely low risk of developing pre-eclampsia in future.

However, the good news is that *most* women who develop pre-eclampsia in a first pregnancy do *not* suffer recurrence. If they have no predisposing medical problems, including kidney disease or chronic hypertension, their risk of a recurrence of severe disease is about 1 in 20—the same level of risk that applies to all first-time mothers. If there are predisposing factors, the odds of suffering severe pre-eclampsia in a second pregnancy rise to around 1 in 10; each time pre-eclampsia recurs it boosts the risk for the next pregnancy.

It is rare, but possible, to have a first brush with pre-eclampsia in a second or later pregnancy. Sometimes this happens after a change of partner, for reasons examined more closely in Chapter 6, but in other cases there is no apparent reason. This is the disease of exceptions, and almost any pattern is possible. For example, a woman may have a normal first pregnancy, a severely affected second pregnancy and then normal later pregnancies, all with the same partner. Or she may follow a pre-eclamptic first pregnancy with one or two normal pregnancies and then suffer an inexplicable recurrence. Pre-eclampsia usually recurs in milder form, but not always, and in rare cases it gets worse with each recurrence. The following case histories give some idea of the diversity of possible patterns of occurrence.

I suffered severe pre-eclampsia in my first pregnancy and was delivered by emergency Caesarean section at 28½ weeks: the baby died after 3 weeks in intensive care. My obstetrician told me that it was quite likely I would suffer from PET in a milder form in my next pregnancy. In fact my second pregnancy and my third were perfectly normal. But in my fourth pregnancy I had a sudden onset of PET at 34 weeks and was delivered by Caesarean 2 days later. My obstetrician was as shocked as I was by the unexpected recurrence.

Maire Ni Riain

My first pregnancy was totally normal with an uncomplicated labour. But in my second pregnancy I noticed swelling of the ankles and fingers at about 31 weeks and suffered nausea and vomiting. My blood pressure was found to be raised and I had protein in my urine. At first I was told to rest at home, but eventually I was admitted to hospital and the baby was delivered at 34 weeks by Caesarean section, after which I had to be weaned off my blood pressure tablets slowly, over about 10 weeks. I still don't know why it occurred in my second pregnancy and not my first and the medical staff were surprised as well. The only difference between the two pregnancies was that the first produced a boy and the second a girl.

Jacqueline Worthington

After a miscarriage at 14 weeks I developed severe pre-eclampsia in my next pregnancy. I had a son after an emergency Caesarean at 29 weeks, who weighed 520 g (just over 1 lb) and lived for 3 days. My next pregnancy followed a very similar pattern, resulting in another Caesarean, this time at 26 weeks. Caroline weighed 590 g and lived for a month. At this stage I still don't know if I'll ever have a family.

Anon.

Pre-eclampsia runs in families, so the sisters and daughters of affected women have an increased risk in their own pregnancies. The clear implication is that pre-eclampsia has a genetic component, although the relevant gene or genes have not yet been identified.

Other factors that may increase a woman's risk of suffering pre-eclampsia include:

- *Increasing age*, particularly after 35;
- *Short stature*;
- *Pre-existing medical conditions*, including chronic hypertension, kidney disease, diabetes, and migraine;
- *Multiple pregnancy*.

The widely-held belief that overweight women are at particular risk is now known to be mistaken. Social class has no bearing on the condition and smoking does not enhance the risk.

Most of the known risk factors apply to the mother. But while her genes and constitution have a lot to do with it, there are some situations where the baby's constitution is also important. This raises the question of whether or not the father contributes to the disease—whether his genes, inherited by the baby, are part of the picture.

The answer to this question is not known (see Chapter 6, p. 132), but there are some situations where the baby, rather than the mother, seems to be the prime mover in the evolution of pre-eclampsia, particularly when there is an abnormally large placenta. We have already mentioned two conditions associated with large placentas that carry an increased risk of pre-eclampsia—hydatidiform mole and multiple pregnancy—but there are others, notably a condition called *placental hydrops*, in which the placenta retains an enormous amount of fluid. Rhesus disease, congenital malformation, and genetic abnormalities can all cause hydropic placentas and increase the risk of pre-eclampsia.

These odd situations may represent the tip of an almost invisible iceberg and it may be that there are many instances of pre-eclampsia where the baby, or more likely its placenta, is the prime cause rather than the mother.

5 · Keeping one step ahead

Although we have dwelt at length on the worst consequences of pre-eclampsia, the truth is that these days such dangerous complications are very much the exception rather than the rule; much of the credit for this achievement belongs to the modern antenatal care programme, which is largely geared to anticipating and neutralizing these dangers.

Of course, any screening programme is only as good as the people providing it, and the fact that a small minority of women suffering from pre-eclampsia continue to slip through its protective net shows the current system is not perfect. But then screening for pre-eclampsia is much more complex than screening for, say, spina bifida, when the definitive signs can be detected at a particular stage of pregnancy. The professionals screening for pre-eclampsia have to contend with an enemy that appears in many different guises, sometimes slowly and with warning, sometimes with devastating speed out of the blue. They have to be ready for an attack at any time in the last 20 weeks of pregnancy, which means there is no 'right time' for testing, and they have to grapple with the paradox that this most treacherous condition is a largely silent enemy, with the victim herself feeling perfectly well—even 'glowing'—and therefore not inclined to believe she has a problem.

These difficulties are compounded by the lack of significant progress in understanding and controlling the disease. As the prime cause of pre-eclampsia is still unknown, there is no way of predicting accurately who is going to suffer from it, no single reliable diagnostic test, no universally effective preventive measure, and no known cure, except to end the pregnancy.

What doctors *should* be able to do is diagnose the disease at an early stage by rigorous screening for the characteristic clinical signs, monitor its progress in both mother and baby, and deliver babies early enough to pre-empt serious illness.

The motto underlying this three-tier protection plan is 'always keep one step ahead of events'.

For convenience, the time course of pre-eclampsia can be divided into four stages, as shown in Table 5.1. The aim of all doctors involved in antenatal screening should be to make the diagnosis in stage one, admit mothers to hospital with the onset of stage two and to deliver their babies before the onset of stage three. Stage four, the perilous final phase, when the mother's systems begin to break down, is a crisis which, in an ideal world, should never be reached.

Table 5.1 The four stages of pre-eclampsia. The table indicates the normal duration of each stage of the pre-eclamptic process, and typical signs and symptoms which might occur at each stage.

	Stage 1 (no protein-uria)	Stage 2 (protein-uric)	Stage 3 (sympto-matic)	Stage 4 (compli-cations)
Typical durations	2 weeks – 3 months	2 days – 3 weeks	2 hours – 3 days	Brief
Hypertension	+	+	+	+
Proteinuria	–	+	+	+
Oedema	+/–	+/–	+/–	+/–
High blood uric acid	++/–	+	+	+
Reduced platelet count	+/–	+/–	++/–	++/–
Abnormal liver tests	+/–	+/–	++/–	++/–
Intrauterine growth retardation	+/–	+/–	+/–	+/–
Symptoms	–	–	+	+
Convulsions, HELLP syndrome, pulmonary oedema, etc.	–	–	–	+

+/–   may occur
++/– usually occurs
+   always or nearly always occurs

In practice, this antenatal safety net enables most susceptible women to run the gauntlet of pre-eclampsia in safety; indeed they are steered past the dangers so effectively that many do not even realize their health was ever at risk.

Ironically, though, antenatal care is now in danger of becoming the victim of its own success. The dangers of pre-eclampsia have not been abolished, merely pushed out of sight, but they are now so well hidden that the apparent justification for routine antenatal checks has largely disappeared. These days most pregnant women —and even some of their carers—do not believe there is much to worry about.

This misconception has led to a very common problem in the management of pre-eclampsia, with the mother unconsciously but persistently undermining the care being offered because she cannot see why it is necessary.

The dangers of pre-eclampsia can only be kept at bay by co-operation between pregnant women and their carers, which is why we now describe in detail how the system works and why it is organized the way it is.

SCREENING FOR PRE-ECLAMPSIA

Although the foundations for pre-eclampsia are laid in the first half of pregnancy, the disease does not normally manifest itself until the second half; so there is a need to screen for pre-eclampsia from 20 weeks.

One of the most critical aspects of screening is the length of the interval between checks. This is difficult to standardize because the disease has an extremely variable speed of progression, with some cases developing over months and others boiling up to danger levels with unnerving speed. In cases of so-called fulminating pre-eclampsia, the mother and her doctors are confronted with a raging crisis, which has evolved from nothing in the space of a week or two, sometimes even less. An interval of more than 2 weeks, or even more than 1 week, between checks can allow such cases to develop undetected.

It is normal practice in the UK for pregnant women to be offered antenatal checks at 20, 24, and 28 weeks, then every 2 weeks to 36 weeks, then every week until full term. But this leaves two potentially dangerous month-long gaps, between 20 and 28 weeks, in which early-onset pre-eclampsia can escape detection, which is why disasters—including maternal deaths—occur more often during this critical period.

I had an antenatal check at 23 weeks and was told everything was fine. My next appointment was arranged for 4 weeks later; but at 24 weeks I began to suffer prolonged bouts of upper abdominal pain and vomiting, which became increasingly severe and frequent over the next 3 weeks.

During this period I saw no fewer than four different doctors—one of them twice!—about the pain, which was variously diagnosed as a 'tummy bug', heartburn, and finally gallstones. But none of them suspected there was any problem with the pregnancy itself and, since I was not yet due for an antenatal check, not one of them offered to take my blood pressure or test my urine.

In fact I was made to feel so confident that the pregnancy was normal that I actually postponed the antenatal check scheduled for 27 weeks to attend my own farewell party at the office. A few days later I began to feel really ill, with headache and a ringing in my ears on top of the ever-present abdominal pain. But in my ignorance I just assumed these were normal 'discomforts' of pregnancy. That night I developed the most appalling pain in the back of my head which would not shift, even with the strong painkillers I was taking for my 'gallstones'.

I had a very disturbed night, and the next morning my husband called the doctor out. This was the first time in the course of the illness that I had seen the doctor who was actually responsible for my antenatal care. When he took my blood pressure—190/125, I believe—he nearly fell through the floor. I had masses of protein in my urine, and he called an ambulance immediately because he thought I was on the verge of having a fit.

My baby was delivered by Caesarean section within a few hours of arriving at the hospital. At first they said they would try to hold on for a few days for the baby's sake, but they decided my condition was too serious to risk any delay. The baby, who weighed only 1 lb 12 oz, was given a 50/50 chance, but his lungs were very immature and he lasted less than 2 days.

I have since been told my case was so bad that even if the illness had been diagnosed earlier the outcome would have been no different. But I can't help thinking that if my antenatal checks had been more frequent, the pregnancy might have lasted long enough for my baby to have had a better chance.

Anon.

To ensure the detection of *all* cases of pre-eclampsia under *all* circumstances, expectant mothers would need to be seen every week from 20 weeks onwards. Clearly this level of care would not be cost-effective for the health service or popular with patients, so doctors compromise by tailoring the frequency of antenatal checks to the perceived risk of pre-eclampsia in individual patients.

However, in practice, it is as difficult for doctors to predict which of their patients is likely to suffer from pre-eclampsia and when the disease will strike as it is for meteorologists to forecast next year's weather!

When women 'book in' for antenatal care at the end of the first trimester, their risk-rating for pre-eclampsia can be roughly categorized as low, medium or high, according to criteria described below, and the pattern of their checks planned accordingly.

In our view, low-risk women need to be screened for the disease every 4 weeks between 20 and 32 weeks and then every 2 weeks up to delivery; medium risk women—which includes all 'untried' first-time mothers—should be screened at 20 and 24 weeks, every 2 weeks to 36 weeks and then every week to delivery, so closing the gap between 24 and 28 weeks. High-risk women need to be seen even more often on a schedule tailored to their individual needs, but that closes the gap between 20 and 24 weeks. However, once a woman in any risk category shows any of the warning signs associated with pre-eclampsia, her risk-rating increases and the intervals between checks must be shortened. As the disease tends to progress increasingly rapidly, the checks must ultimately become so frequent that they can only be carried out in hospital.

Estimating your risk

The factors that increase a woman's susceptibility to pre-eclampsia were described in Chapter 4 (see p. 88). For example, all women in their first pregnancy must be rated medium risk, because as many as 1 in 20 will develop severe pre-eclampsia. If a first-time mother is 'elderly' (over 40), has a pre-existing medical problem such as chronic hypertension or kidney disease, is expecting more than one baby or has any of the other additional risk factors listed on page 000, she moves automatically into the high-risk group.

Women who have suffered multiple or particularly severe attacks of pre-eclampsia in previous pregnancies are also rated high-risk. The typical low-risk mother is aged 25–35, is in her second or third pregnancy after a normal preceding pregnancy or pregnancies and is in good general health. But these estimates of risk are very crude and cannot be applied accurately to individuals with any degree of certainty.

Antenatal tests

The main problem with diagnosing pre-eclampsia is that because its origins are obscure there is no specific diagnostic test which can provide a 'yes/no' answer to the question: 'Does this woman have pre-eclampsia?'.

Until such time as it is more fully understood, pre-eclampsia must remain a 'syndrome', recognized not by its unique causal agent but by a collection of characteristic signs and symptoms, which can each have other causes taken individually, but usually indicate pre-eclampsia when they occur together.

Once the pattern of antenatal care has been determined, four basic tests need to be repeated at each visit to detect the warning signs of pre-eclampsia. At least two signs must be present before the diagnosis can be made. The tests include:

(1) blood pressure measurement;

(2) weight check;

(3) assessment of the baby's growth by the size of the uterus;

(4) urine test for protein.

Blood pressure

Although a rise in blood pressure is usually the first sign of pre-eclampsia, it is an unreliable one, partly because blood pressure is naturally variable, with alternating 'highs' and 'lows', and partly because the measurement technique itself is rather crude and inaccurate. One high reading alone is not necessarily significant—the readings must be consistently raised. The actual level of the blood pressure is probably less important than the amount by which it has risen above a 'baseline' measurement taken in early pregnancy. A reading of 140/90, for example, would be high if the baseline reading was 90/60, but not if it was 130/80. Any reading 25–30 mmHg higher than the baseline measurement should be taken seriously—the systolic (upper) figure is as important in this respect as the diastolic figure. Even a high reading may not mean pre-eclampsia. As explained in Chapter 3 (p. 34), it is common for the blood pressure to fall in early pregnancy then climb back to normal levels towards term. If a woman's normal blood pressure is on the high side—which will not be known if her blood pressure has been measured for the first time in pregnancy—this gradual return to pre-pregnant levels can mimic the onset of pre-eclampsia.

A very extreme example of this phenomenon was reported in America in 1947. A woman first seen in her second pregnancy at 34 weeks had slightly raised blood pressure of 140/90, which rose further to 140/95 in labour. Six weeks after delivery, her blood pressure had shot up to 190/120. The woman was observed through four subsequent pregnancies and a recurrent pattern was noted. Between pregnancies her blood pressure ranged from 180/105 to 280/160; it fell dramatically in early pregnancy to reach a low of 110/60, then climbed back towards her normal levels in the final month. This case shows how pregnancy can conceal chronic hypertension and how the reappearance of chronic hypertension can be mistaken for pre-eclampsia.

The classic 'cluster' of diagnostic signs is high blood pressure combined with protein in the urine, but even this can be misleading.

A misleading case of apparent pre-eclampsia

Mrs E disliked doctors and hospitals and in her first pregnancy did her best to avoid antenatal care. When seen in hospital at almost 20 weeks her blood pressure was normal at 130/80, but she managed to slip away before providing a urine sample. The same thing occurred when she saw her own GP a month later. Four weeks later, when her blood pressure was slightly raised at 150/85, the GP insisted on seeing a urine sample, which was found to contain three 'plusses' of protein.

Mrs E was admitted to hospital with what seemed to be proteinuric pre-eclampsia, although no one could tell whether or not the proteinuria was a new development because there were no previous urine samples to refer to.

Mrs E remained in hospital, for the next 9 weeks, apparently suffering from severe pre-eclampsia. The diagnosis became increasingly uncertain because there was no deterioration in her condition and no sign of problems for the baby. However, she was advised to stay in hospital, where she was induced and delivered without complication at nearly 38 weeks.

After delivery the proteinuria persisted and Mrs E's blood pressure remained elevated. Her doctors eventually decided that she was suffering from chronic kidney disease and chronic mild hypertension and had never had pre-eclampsia. As she refused further investigation, a definitive diagnosis was never made.

This case shows, among other things, how apparent warning signs can only be interpreted with accuracy if they can be compared with 'baseline' measurements taken in early pregnancy. Lack of co-operation by Mrs E led to 9 weeks hospitalization, which could probably have been avoided had she complied with normal antenatal care.

Oedema

Oedema is probably the most confusing of all possible signs of pre-eclampsia because it is a common and even desirable feature of normal pregnancy. However, swelling is suspicious if it is associated with weight gain of more than 1 kg (2.2 lb) per week, particularly if the blood pressure is up.

Slow fetal growth

Slow fetal growth is not usually thought of as a sign of pre-eclampsia, but it can indicate a failing placenta which, as explained in Chapter 4 (p. 55), appears to be the source of the disease. Slow growth is likely to be suspected if the uterus feels smaller than it should, and can be confirmed by ultrasound measurement of the girth of the baby's abdomen. However, even this measurement is not helpful unless the pregnancy has been accurately dated because the baby's size must be assessed in relation to its maturity. This is why doctors are so keen to establish the true time of conception at the beginning of pregnancy.

Uric acid levels

One additional test that is sometimes useful to confirm a diagnosis of pre-eclampsia is a check on blood levels of the waste product uric acid. A rising concentration, showing that the kidneys are not working as well as they should, can be an early sign of pre-eclampsia which predates the appearance of protein in the urine.

None of these screening tests can reveal the underlying problem in the placenta; at best they merely show up its reflected effects in mother and baby, and while these reflections sometimes provide a clear picture, they can also distort the truth and mislead the observer.

To employ another image, screening for pre-eclampsia is like trying to find out what is going on inside a house by looking through

the windows but never going inside. What doctors see depends on
the window they choose to look through. If they restrict themselves
to only one or two windows they are likely to get an incomplete
impression. They may think all is well simply because they have
failed to look through the right window into the room where all
the trouble is brewing.

In summary then, just as the presence of only one sign of pre-
eclampsia is never enough to make a diagnosis, so the absence of
any one sign never excludes the diagnosis with certainty. There is
no simple formula and medical staff must maintain a constant, wary
vigilance.

COMMON DIAGNOSTIC MISTAKES

Blood pressure

The most common mistake, in which mothers often collude with
doctors, is to discount a raised blood pressure and ascribe it to
'nervousness'. As hypertension is usually the first sign of pre-
eclampsia, and as pre-eclampsia is such a dangerous disease, no-one
can afford to be this complacent. A high reading should *never* be
ignored, although it may turn out to be a false alarm in the end.
This applies to systolic as well as diastolic readings: a blood pressure
of 160/80 needs to be taken as seriously as one of 140/90.

Proteinuria

Another common error is to underestimate the importance of testing
for proteinuria. A urine test is sometimes not carried out, or the
result is not recorded, if a doctor has no reason to suspect problems.
This is an unacceptable omission because proteinuria can accompany
only slightly raised blood pressure or even *predate* a rise in blood
pressure. When protein is found in the urine it is not uncommon
for doctors to play down its significance, particularly if it is associated with only moderate hypertension; such cases may be labelled
'mild pre-eclampsia' whereas in fact *all* proteinuric pre-eclampsia
should be regarded as severe.

At 21 weeks I started vomiting at nights. In between bouts of vomiting
I was hardly able to lie down because of the pain in my upper abdomen.

This happened on about six occasions over a period of 13 days, until eventually I was admitted to hospital with suspected pre-eclampsia.

I was kept in hospital for two nights, but because I did not have a vomiting bout they—and I—thought I had recovered. My blood pressure was apparently normal, but I was swollen and exhausted. The night I was sent home I had another vomiting attack, and we drove straight back to the hospital, where I was admitted and monitored again.

The following morning (Christmas Day—definitely not a time to be ill!) I was discharged despite the fact that my card was marked 'protein $++++$', which I now know is extremely high.

The following night I was again very ill, but we waited until the next morning to ensure that we saw my own doctor. He immediately had me admitted to hospital, although he had to argue with the registrar on the 'phone.

At first I was treated as though there was nothing the matter with me, but that changed when I started experiencing visual disturbances like flashing disco lights. When the consultant said 'We've got to finish this pregnancy to save your life,' I just thought 'Thank God somebody is doing something for me at last'.

My baby was delivered stillborn at 23 weeks, and I was so ill that I stayed in intensive care for 3 days and needed an oxygen mask for several days longer.

I felt increasingly angry as I recovered and could think clearly about how I had been treated. The excuse was always that I had developed pre-eclampsia so early in pregnancy and that I didn't appear to have consistently high blood pressure. I feel the loss of my daughter and the seriousness of my own condition was a direct result of their refusal to take appropriate action.

Pam Clark

Abdominal pain, vomiting, and jaundice

The significance of abdominal pain and vomiting is also often missed, particularly by family doctors who encounter such symptoms every day in their non-pregnant patients, and jaundice is a rare presentation of pre-eclampsia, which is frequently misinterpreted.

The hidden complications

Finally, many doctors still fail to look for the hidden complications of pre-eclampsia, which are generally more serious than 'visible' signs like hypertension and proteinuria. This is particularly true of

liver and blood clotting disturbances in the mother and problems
with the baby's growth and oxygen supply.

All these mistakes have a common root: failure to find out what is
going on in the house of pre-eclampsia by looking through all the
available windows.

THE CRUCIAL TIMING OF ADMISSION

The point of admitting pre-eclamptic women to hospital is not always
clear, even to doctors themselves. Patients are often told they are being
admitted for 'bed rest' to bring down their blood pressure. This is
clearly nonsense. No-one could seriously argue that hospitals are con-
ducive to rest, with no privacy, constant noise and bustle, and hard,
narrow beds. In any case, the blood pressure is not the fundamental
problem in pre-eclampsia, it is merely one outward signal of a complex, multifaceted disease. The true justification for admitting
women to hospital is to keep one step ahead of events by rigorous
monitoring. As pre-eclampsia advances it becomes ever more unstable,
so that checks on its progress need to be carried out more and more frequently until eventually this surveillance can only be maintained in hospital; and not just any old hospital, but one with the resources to deliver
within the hour if a major emergency flares up.

The timing of admission is crucial. Stage three pre-eclampsia,
when the mother has begun to feel ill, and eclampsia itself, are both
emergencies that justify admission by the local flying squad—a team
of specialists who personally conduct pregnant women to hospital by
ambulance.

If new proteinuria (+ or more) is detected, together with hypertension, however mild, the woman must be assumed to be in stage
2 (proteinuric) pre-eclampsia. This stage is so unstable that her
safety cannot be guaranteed for the next 24 hours and she should
be admitted to hospital on the same day. Failure to admit at this
stage is one of the most common causes of preventable obstetric
disasters.

The cost of ignoring proteinuria

Mrs F was just before term at the end of an uneventful first pregnancy
when her diastolic blood pressure rose to 85 mmHg. A trace of protein in

the urine at that time became a definite 'plus' 1 week later and this result was confirmed by a further test 3 days after that. Throughout this time the diastolic pressure remained at 85.

Although Mrs F was by now beyond her due date, admission for induction was not arranged. However, 6 days later, now at nearly 42 weeks, her diastolic pressure rose to 100 and the proteinuria had increased to '+++'. She was admitted and induced, delivering a good-sized daughter. Her labour was uncomplicated, although she needed one injection of hydralazine to control her blood pressure.

A few hours after delivery she lost about a pint of blood from her vagina and a large amount of blood accumulated around her episiotomy stitches. Mrs F's doctors attempted to drain the blood away but any new incision or suture immediately stimulated fresh bleeding because, as was later discovered, her clotting system had ceased to work properly. Blood transfusions were started and the obstetrician set about controlling the slow but continuous bleeding. By the time he had finished Mrs F had been under general anaesthesia for more than 3½ hours and had received several pints of blood and blood substitute.

When Mrs F came round she found she could not see clearly and examination revealed that the retinae of both eyes had become detached—a well-known, but fortunately rare complication of severe pre-eclampsia. The next day she needed another 5 pints of blood to replace the full amount she had lost.

Happily both retinae reattached themselves so that by 6 weeks after delivery normal sight was almost fully restored.

In this case proteinuric pre-eclampsia was associated with mild hypertension but severe clotting problems. No-one can say for sure, but it is highly likely that if Mrs F had been admitted as soon as proteinuria was detected, she could have been spared the serious complications that ensued.

In some cases, a diagnosis of proteinuric pre-eclampsia will prove mistaken and the woman can be allowed home, but this is a dangerous option if the diagnosis is confirmed, however apparently stable the patient's condition: she is now committed to staying in hospital until delivery.

The development of mild to moderate hypertension on its own is not a reason for admission but it does indicate the need for more frequent monitoring, and some doctors like to admit hypertensive patients to hospital for a day or two just to assess the extent of the problem. After that they can be monitored in a well-organized day care unit, working in collaboration with GPs and community midwives, unless and until more ominous signs appear.

WHEN TO DELIVER

If the health and safety of the baby were not so important then every woman with pre-eclampsia would be delivered as soon as the condition was diagnosed because, once it gains a toehold, pre-eclampsia invariably gets worse and does not begin to regress until after delivery. So there are no advantages—and plenty of risks—for the mother in allowing the pregnancy to continue.

However, babies of less than 8 months maturity are generally better off inside the womb than out, as long as they themselves are not being seriously affected by pre-eclampsia. So delivery before this stage may help the mother but harm her baby, and the more premature the baby, the higher the risk.

The most agonizing dilemmas for doctors and parents arise when severe pre-eclampsia occurs before 26 weeks, when delivery is best for the mother but will almost certainly kill the baby. Such tragic but necessary sacrifices leave dreadful emotional scars. Fortunately, rapid improvements in the care of premature babies have made these situations quite rare nowadays. Thirty years ago, a premature baby's survival was only a remote possibility before 32 weeks, and even up to 34 weeks its chances were very slim. But today babies delivered at 32 weeks or later can be expected to thrive and develop normally and many born earlier—even, in a few cases, as early as 26 weeks — survive and do well thanks to the skilled treatment they receive in special care nurseries.

When making decisions about delivery, therefore, doctors take into account the maturity of the pregnancy as well as the severity of the disease. A woman with mild (non-proteinuric) pre-eclampsia would undoubtedly be kept going if the problem appeared at, say, 28 weeks, but might be delivered if it appeared at 38 weeks, by which time a baby is fully mature. With a woman suffering from severe (proteinuric) pre-eclampsia, whose condition could deteriorate at any time into a life-threatening crisis there would have to be very good reasons for continuing the pregnancy, beyond 34–36 weeks, although before this time delivery might be delayed to allow the baby a little more time to mature. However, if a woman's systems are under so much strain that she is feeling ill or has even suffered an eclamptic convulsion, immediate delivery is the *only* option, *whatever* the stage of the pregnancy.

Even in situations where the mother's condition is stable enough to enable her to continue with the pregnancy, delivery is sometimes necessary for the baby's sake. The sick placenta may be keeping the baby so short of food and/or oxygen that delivery offers the best chance of survival. It is common for the mother's condition to reflect the baby's situation, but sometimes there is a mismatch and the baby may be critically ill while its mother is relatively well, or vice versa. So assessing how well the baby is coping in the womb is a vital aspect of deciding when to deliver.

MONITORING THE BABY'S HEALTH

Pre-eclampsia is a shared disease and, once it is diagnosed, regular checks must be carried out on the baby as well as the mother. Sometimes the baby's problems are detected before the mother's condition becomes apparent—for example, if a hitherto active baby becomes sluggish and still—although it normally happens the other way round.

The basic tool for checking on the baby's well-being is the cardio-tocograph or CTG—known in the United States as the *non-stress test* (NST). As described in Chapter 3 (p. 47), this records the pattern of the baby's heartbeat, which is directly affected by the oxygen shortage associated with pre-eclampsia. Doctors checking the read-ings (traces) from these tests look for three particular warning signs:

Absence of 'accelerations'

Absence of the accelerations in the heart rate which normally occur when the baby is in an active phase is one of the warning signs. This implies that the baby is drowsier than usual, but is very rarely a cause for anxiety unless combined with one or both of the other signs.

'Decelerations'

Decelerations in the heart rate, usually coinciding with maternal 'tightenings', or Braxton Hicks contractions, indicate that the baby is becoming distressed when the uterus contracts, although it recovers quickly afterwards. Such a baby will almost certainly not be able to cope with the much greater stress of labour and needs to be monitored very closely in future, although immediate delivery is not necessary unless the decelerations are combined with loss of variability.

'Loss of variability'

Loss of variability—the absence of the second-by-second fluctuations in the heart rate, which are signs of healthy brain activity—results in a 'flat' trace. This is the most serious warning sign, a true SOS signal from a baby in extreme distress requiring urgent delivery.

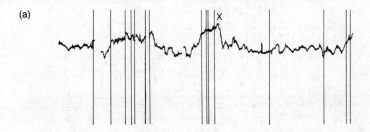

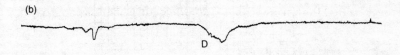

Fig. 5.1 Fetal heart rate patterns in normal and pre-eclamptic pregnancy. (a) A normal cardiotocograph (CTG). The horizontal line shows fluctuations in the fetal heart rate. An acceleration, marked by a cross, is associated with fetal movements, recorded by the mother and marked by the vertical lines on the trace. (b) A severely abnormal cardiotocograph. The horizontal line shows no accelerations, a deceleration (marked 'D'), and an absence of the variations in rate which are characteristic of good health. Babies showing this pattern die unless delivered urgently.

The major limitation of a CTG test is that it tells doctors only how the baby is *now*, not how it will be tomorrow, let alone next week. So the test is useful only when the situation is bad enough to justify at least daily monitoring. In such circumstances there is no doubt that the test prevents many many deaths *in utero* by indicating the

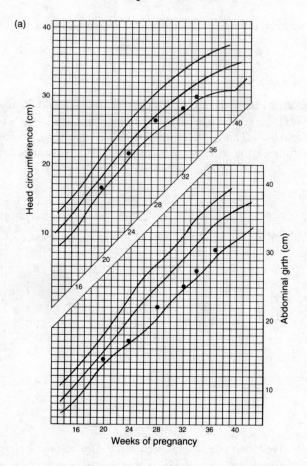

Fig. 5.2 (a)　Ultrasound measurements of fetal growth. The charts record measurements of head circumference (above) and abdominal girth (below). The middle line in each chart shows the average rate of growth, and the upper and lower lines record the limits of normality. The chart shows normal growth in a naturally small baby who weighed 5 lb 9 oz when born at 38 weeks.

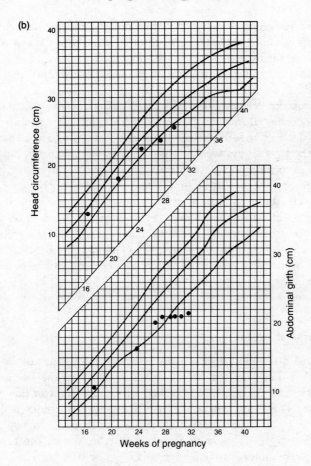

Fig. 5.2 (b)   Ultrasound measurements of fetal growth. The chart shows growth retardation from around 27 weeks in a baby affected by severe pre-eclampsia. The growth of the abdomen was more affected than that of the head, which is not unusual. After delivery, at 31–32 weeks, this baby weighed 2 lb 1 oz.

need for pre-emptive delivery. Before the test became available it was impossible to predict which babies were likely to die as a result of their problems. After this test was introduced in Oxford in 1975, the stillbirth rate for women with very severe pre-eclampsia dropped six-fold.

Doctors' knowledge of the baby's well-being can be supplemented by other tests, all involving the use of ultrasound. For example, the baby's size and growth rate can be estimated from measurements of its girth. It is always worrying if a baby is unduly small, but less so if it is continuing to grow at a normal rate. However, if a baby stops growing or, worse, becomes thinner, there is much more cause for anxiety about its chances of further survival in the womb.

The trouble with growth rate measurements is that it takes time to see the trends clearly. Accurate measurements taken by skilled operators can be useful if repeated at a maximum frequency of once a week over several weeks. But while this enables doctors to detect and monitor a slowly-developing problem, it cannot reveal acute difficulties.

Biophysical profile

A skilled ultrasound operator can do much more than just *measure* the baby. The way the baby lies and moves and the volume of amniotic fluid in which it is bathed all provide clues to how well the baby is feeling, which is why a worrying CTG result is often followed by a comprehensive ultrasound assessment, known as a *biophysical profile*. This helps to reveal whether or not the baby is likely to die unless delivered urgently.

The biophysical profile is a technique for 'scoring' the ultrasound picture of the baby in the womb. A maximum score of two is awarded for each of the following features:

- breathing movements;
- limb movements;
- good posture (a comfortable, curled up position);
- adequate amniotic fluid.

Any feature judged to be abnormal attracts a zero score. The best possible score is 8/8—or 10/10 if the pattern of the heartbeat is included. A score of zero indicates a very sick baby, needing urgent delivery to save its life. A score of 2 or 4 would normally justify delivery unless the baby were premature; a score of 6 or 8 would not call for action but would need to be rechecked within 12–24 hours.

Doppler ultrasound measurement

The relatively new technique of Doppler ultrasound measurement of blood flow patterns (see p. 50), which is being slowly introduced in maternity units, can give early warning of impending troubles for the baby before the CTG becomes abnormal. It is most helpful when used to measure the speed of flow through the arteries of the umbilical cord. A loss or reversal of flow when the baby's heart is between beats is a sign that the circulation through the placenta is abnormal (see Fig. 5.3). This means that problems may build up and early delivery may be necessary in future, so regular monitoring is necessary.

TREATMENT OPTIONS

Delivery

At present the only effective treatment for pre-eclampsia is delivery. This is usually advantageous for both mother and baby, but in some early cases the needs of mother and baby are in direct conflict—the mother at risk of dangerous complications if delivery does not take place and the baby at risk of extreme prematurity if it does.

In circumstances like these it is desirable to hold on for as long as possible, and sometimes doctors can buy a little more time for the baby by controlling the mother's blood pressure. Hypertension is the consequence not the cause of pre-eclampsia, so controlling the blood pressure does not solve the problem or make the sick placenta any healthier. But it can reduce the risk of third-stage complications and so enable a blighted pregnancy to continue for a little longer.

Controlling blood pressure

Severe hypertension threatens the small arteries of the body, particularly in the brain, with forces they cannot cope with, and in extreme cases this can lead to death from cerebral haemorrhage. The threshold at which pressure-induced arterial injury occurs is

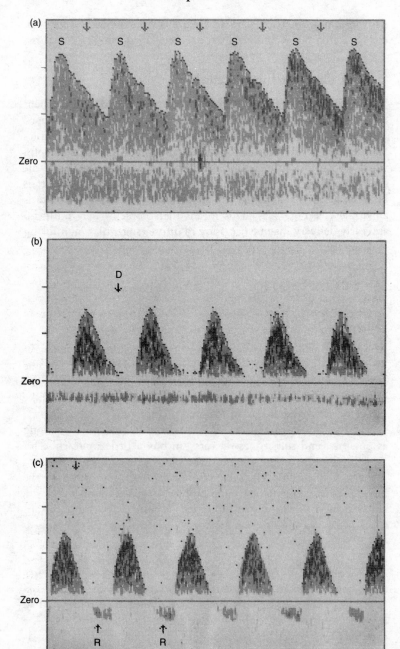

extremely high, although it varies from individual to individual; but once this threshold is crossed, dangerous situations develop very rapidly. At such critical moments the use of drugs to control the blood pressure is a life-saving measure, although never more than a temporary expedient.

In previous generations, the raised blood pressure of pre-eclampsia was ascribed to anxiety and/or over-activity and treated by heavy sedation. Although the use of sedative drugs to treat hypertension was shown to be ineffective as long ago as the 1950s, the habit persisted until the early 1980s. However, the antihypertensive drugs most commonly used today have more direct effects on the circulatory system.

There is no absolute rule about the level of blood pressure at which treatment should be started, but most doctors agree that pressures at or above 170/110 should be controlled. Some doctors begin treatment at lower levels of blood pressure and a very few specialists go to the opposite extreme, rarely prescribing antihypertensive drugs at all, despite the known risks of uncontrolled hypertension. These doctors believe that the high blood pressure of pre-eclampsia is nature's way of maintaining a good blood flow to the placenta through an increasingly obstructed circulation and that by reducing the blood pressure they would risk damaging the baby's supply line. But this is a minority view which has never been substantiated.

Antihypertensive agents used in pre-eclampsia fall into two categories: fast-acting drugs for short-term control in emergencies, and slower-acting agents, which can maintain control in a more sustained fashion.

Fig. 5.3 Doppler measurements of fetal blood flow in normal and pre-eclamptic pregnancy. In each case the shaded area above the zero line records the pulsed flow in one artery of the umbilical cord, while the shaded area below the line records flow in the vein. 'S' marks peak flow during each beat of the baby's heart and the arrows mark the decline in flow between beats. In (a) (a normal baby) the flow of blood never stops, even between beats; in (b), a baby affected by pre-eclampsia, the pattern is the same as in (a), but blood flow stops between the heartbeats (marked by 'D'); in (c), a severely-compromised baby, flow does not merely halt between beats but bounces back in reverse (marked by 'R'), shown by the shaded areas below the zero line.

Fast-acting antihypertensive drugs

Pre-eclampsia may develop so rapidly and with such severity that it is vital to bring down the blood pressure as quickly as possible. The drug most commonly used in this situation is *hydralazine*, which dilates the arteries, lowers their resistance to blood flow and so reduces the blood pressure, sometimes very dramatically. Although hydralazine is very effective, it causes unpleasant side-effects, including severe headache, palpitations, restlessness, and anxiety, in about half the people who use it. These side-effects tend to mimic the symptoms of impending eclampsia, which can be extremely confusing for doctors. Another disadvantage of hydralazine is that has to be administered by injection—usually a continuous infusion into an arm vein, which is not very convenient.

Alternative fast-acting drugs include a group called *calcium channel blockers*, which also work by dilating blood vessels. One of these drugs, *nifedipine*, acts more rapidly when taken by mouth than hydralazine does when given directly into a vein. It also causes fewer side-effects, although headaches, unfortunately, are even more common.

These drugs are primarily given for the acute relief of high blood pressure, but pre-eclamptic hypertension must be controlled for a few days at least, and often for longer, so the effects of fast-acting treatment must be reinforced by medication that lowers the blood pressure in a more sustained way. Here the choice lies between methyldopa and a group of drugs collectively known as 'beta-blockers'.

Slower-acting antihypertensive drugs

Methyldopa, which works by suppressing the hypertensive activity of the sympathetic nervous system, can control blood pressure within 6–12 hours when given in adequate doses, but it tends to cause extreme sleepiness for the first 48 hours and fatigue after that. In fact, methyldopa is rather an old-fashioned drug, although it continues to be used in pregnancy because it appears to be very safe for the baby as well as the mother. The baby shares in the initial sedation and may be temporarily more sluggish, but no serious adverse effects have yet been discovered. This does not necessarily mean other antihypertensives are more risky, but methyldopa is the only blood pressure drug that has been thoroughly tested for use in pregnancy and whose long-term safety for the baby has been established.

Beta-blocking drugs also work by interfering with sympathetic nervous system activity, and cause fewer side-effects than methyldopa. Although their safety in pregnancy has not been so exhaustively investigated, their short-term safety for babies is well established. *Oxprenolol* and *labetalol* work faster than *atenolol* and there have even been claims, which a follow-up study failed to confirm, that oxprenolol promotes fetal growth.

It is a common feature of normal pregnancy for blood pressure to rise progressively during the first 5 days after delivery. This trend may be exaggerated in pre-eclamptic women, so that the highest readings of all occur 5–7 days after delivery. Sometimes other signs and symptoms, including abdominal (liver) pain and even eclampsia, appear for the first time at this stage, which is why it is vitally important not to discharge pre-eclamptic women too early.

Hypertension after delivery needs to be managed in the same way as before, although beta-blockers are preferable to methyldopa because they do not cause sleepiness. Patients can normally be discharged 6–8 days after delivery and antihypertensive treatment reduced or stopped within 2–3 weeks of discharge.

PREVENTION AND CONTROL OF ECLAMPSIA

Eclamptic fits can be prevented by a class of drugs known as anticonvulsants, although the main dilemma for doctors is who to treat—it can be extraordinarily difficult to predict which women are likely to suffer fits.

There are few, if any, reliable signs of impending convulsions. The level of blood pressure is not a useful guide and neither are the degree of proteinuria and the extent of oedema. In fact, the best indicator is a subjective one—how the woman herself *feels*. If she seems entirely well it is most unlikely that she is about to have a fit, but headaches, vomiting or 'epigastric' (upper abdominal) pain are all ominous complaints. The trouble is that because these are non-specific symptoms they can be attributed to comparatively minor problems, like gastroenteritis or 'flu. A diagnostic error like this is unlikely if the woman is already being monitored in hospital, but it is a potential trap for GPs who are not necessarily expecting trouble.

Some obstetricians sidestep the dilemma of whom to treat by prescribing anticonvulsants for all women with proteinuric pre-eclampsia. But this comprehensive approach is not desirable because of the risk of side-effects, which can include excessive—even danger-ous—sedation of mother and baby.

It should be possible to treat women more selectively, but this requires skill and experience and the problem is that, because eclampsia is so rare nowadays, few doctors have wide experience of dealing with the problem. That is why there is a need for specialist centres, to which cases of very severe pre-eclampsia and eclampsia could be referred so that at least some teams of doctors could gain wide experience of the problems involved (see Chapter 7, p. 146).

The overriding aim of good care must be to prevent fits, but this aim is obviously not being realized at present, because statistics on maternal death show that in half of all fatal cases the first eclamptic convulsion occurs *after* admission to a consultant unit. This means one of two things: either the women who are likely to have con-vulsions are not being correctly identified or the treatment given is ineffective.

Anticonvulsant drugs

Drugs like *diazepam* (Valium) or *chlormethiazole* (Heminevrin) are excellent for stopping convulsions quickly, if given in high doses by intravenous infusion, but such doses cause heavy sedation. In many maternity units, these drugs are also used to prevent fits, but the resulting sedation, which may need to be prolonged for 2 or 3 days, also affects the baby after delivery, which is a serious drawback.

A relatively recent alternative for preventing eclamptic con-vulsions is *phenytoin*, a well-tried antiepileptic drug with the advan-tage of causing little sedation.

Another contender is *magnesium sulphate* (see p. 18), a prep-aration that is widely used in the United States for preventing fits. Magnesium sulphate has no sedative effects, which is an advantage for mother and baby, and, although no-one yet knows how it works —despite the fact that it has been in use for more than 50 years— magnesium sulphate appears to be safe and effective in skilled hands.

It has never been a popular treatment in the UK, but this may change in time—and indeed moves are currently afoot to set up a UK trial of magnesium sulphate in preventing eclampsia.

All of these anticonvulsant treatments have a high failure rate and, even when they work, the risk of further fits is high, so they do not obviate the need for urgent delivery.

Once a woman has suffered one or more fits, a major medical emergency is under way. Because it is not possible to breathe during convulsions, the first priority is to prevent suffocation by clearing the airway and giving oxygen. If fitting persists it may be necessary to paralyse the woman, intubate the airway, and put her on a ventilator.

The next priority is to stop the fits with the appropriate medication, such as diazepam injections into a vein, and prevent further convulsions with phenytoin (in the UK) or magnesium sulphate (in the US).

Once the fits have been stopped, the priorities are to control the blood pressure (if necessary), to assess how disturbed the mother's systems are and how the baby is coping, and then deliver the baby as quickly and as safely as possible.

Before, during, and after delivery doctors and midwives have to maintain extreme vigilance and care until all the dangers are clearly on the wane.

INTENSIVE CARE FOR CRISIS MANAGEMENT

In the most serious cases of pre-eclampsia or eclampsia—when individual systems of the body can break down completely—mothers sometimes need to be referred to intensive care units, which specialize in crisis management.

In these circumstances, facilities for supporting breathing with ventilators, monitoring the circulation to the heart with catheters and, if necessary, boosting a failing circulation with drugs can make the difference between life and death.

I was induced a week past my due date because of high blood pressure. The first fit occurred a few hours after delivery, while I was asleep. Afterwards I went into a coma for 3 days and was looked after in intensive care, attached to numerous tubes. When eventually I came round, I was told I had been very seriously ill and it had been touch and go whether I'd survive. I was

advised to avoid a second pregnancy and agreed because the whole experience was so frightening. It took me over a year to recover fully.

Gillian Samuel

Not all doctors agree on the best ways to 'ride the storm' of very
severe pre-eclampsia; and the most controversial aspect of intensive
care is how to manage the maldistribution of fluid within the body,
which the affected woman registers as oedema.

Some experts believe that the reduced circulating blood volume,
which is a classic feature of pre-eclampsia, is a prime cause of such
complications as liver and kidney failure, and seek to expand the
blood volume by giving infusions of fluid. However, others argue
that as the reduced blood volume and the fluid retention in the
tissues probably result from abnormal leakiness in the small blood
vessels, any extra fluid infused into the bloodstream will quickly
leak out into the tissues in the same way, aggravating the oedema
and increasing the risk of complications.

As the kidneys are especially vulnerable to the ravages of pre-
eclampsia, it is standard practice in serious cases to monitor urine
flow with a catheter placed in the bladder. *Anuria*—complete cessation of urine flow—invariably signals kidney failure, and *oliguria*
—a marked reduction in flow—can be ominous, although it may
be a normal response to poor fluid intake, the stress of surgery or
the effects of antihypertensive treatment.

In some cases, oliguria is a sign of a failing circulation. If this is
suspected, the circulation to the heart needs to be monitored by
means of a *central venous pressure* (CVP) line, which is threaded along
an arm or neck vein until the tip reaches the right side of the heart,
where all veins drain. If the central venous pressure is too low, the
heart is not receiving enough blood to work properly and a transfusion may be needed.

One of the most perilous complications of severe pre-eclampsia is
pulmonary oedema, when the airspaces in the lungs fill up with fluid
and the mother begins literally to drown. This crisis is made worse
by kidney failure, which forces the body to retain still more fluid.
In such an emergency, diuretic drugs, which stimulate even severely
weakened kidneys to produce copious urine, may be prescribed and
the mother's breathing may need temporary support from a ventilator until the problem is under control.

A case of pulmonary oedema

Twenty-one weeks into her first pregnancy, Mrs G suddenly began to gain excessive weight; although her blood pressure was normal, a urine test showed three 'plusses' of protein. A week later she was admitted to hospital in the early hours of the morning with abdominal pain, oedema and severe hypertension. Tests revealed such severe disturbances of her liver and clotting system that the pregnancy had to be terminated immediately by Caesarean section, even though Mrs G's extremely premature baby had no chance of survival.

After delivery, a catheter was left in Mrs G's bladder to drain urine continuously. Suddenly, 6 hours after delivery, the flow almost stopped and, at the same time, Mrs G became distressed and breathless. Numerous cracking, bubbling noises could be heard in her chest through a stethoscope as she breathed—a sure sign of free fluid percolating through the air spaces of her lungs. A chest X-ray confirmed the diagnosis of pulmonary oedema.

As Mrs G struggled for breath, she turned blue from lack of oxygen, which had to be supplied through a face mask. She was given diuretics to help her kidneys excrete the surplus fluid and transferred to intensive care in case she needed to be supported on a ventilator.

Fortunately Mrs G managed—just—without a ventilator, but the breathlessness persisted for another three days, after which she rapidly recovered. The evidence in her case suggested that the rapid leakage of blood fluid into her lungs had deprived her kidneys of the fluid they needed to maintain urine output.

Clotting disturbances

Also fraught with danger are the clotting disturbances of severe pre-eclampsia which, at worse, can lead to the widespread, uncontrolled clotting problem known as disseminated intravascular coagulation (DIC, p. 73). The only remedy for DIC, as for all the other third-stage complications of pre-eclampsia, is to deliver the baby. However, as the effect of DIC is to rob the blood of its clotting factors, any major bleeding—and bleeding is a routine complication of delivery—may provoke a life-threatening emergency. It is possible to delay delivery until a fresh supply of clotting factors can be given via transfusion, but this can make matters worse, by providing the fuel for further uncontrolled clotting. The only way out of this desperate situation is to deliver the baby, maintain the circulation as adequately as possible with transfusions, and pray that the natural forces of recovery will do the rest.

THE PSYCHOLOGY OF PRE-ECLAMPSIA

In the early stages of pre-eclampsia it is impossible to forecast how far—and how quickly—the condition will deteriorate. Each new patient may be the one who ends up wracked by convulsions, bleeding uncontrollably or drowning with pulmonary oedema. So each has to be managed and monitored in the same thorough and cautious way.

Naturally, women who have suffered severely in a previous pregnancy need no persuading about the potential gravity of their condition and the need for stringent precautions, but others may not be so compliant. Most are ignorant of the dangers of pre-eclampsia and some have never even *heard* of it. Many have been led to expect that healthy women have normal pregnancies and, since they tend to feel perfectly well at the time of diagnosis, may find it difficult to accept the facts. Sadly, this means that obstetricians are forced to spend a lot of their time arguing with patients who cannot see the need for all the fuss. Of course, this does not always happen, and many women comply readily with what is being done to help them, but it is a common and continuing problem. How do you persuade people to accept surveillance or treatment when they do not believe there is anything wrong with them?

Unfortunately, all the uncertainties about pre-eclampsia described in previous chapters serve to reinforce this dilemma: doctors tend to be vague about what exactly is wrong and why, they cannot say what will happen, they do not offer treatment as such—only time-consuming, inconvenient, and seemingly aimless monitoring. Some doctors undermine their patients' trust still further by saying they want to admit them 'just for a few days', then refusing to allow them home. In fact most women admitted with pre-eclampsia need to stay in hospital until after delivery—which can mean weeks or even, in rare cases, months; and most will be delivered early, not allowed to wait for spontaneous labour at full term.

When I was admitted at 33 weeks I was told I would probably only have to stay a couple of days, so I felt quite calm and relaxed. Then I was told I would have to stay another couple of days to complete some more 24-hour urine collections, although no-one explained what they were for. The day before the baby was delivered, the fetal monitor showed a dip in activity. I was then seen by the senior registrar, who examined me, said: 'You're having a Caesarean in the morning,' and left. I was shocked by the bluntness of the statement and began to cry. If I hadn't cried I don't think anyone would have come to explain things properly to me. I felt angry that up until that point no-one had given any indication that my baby might have to be delivered early. I felt they thought 'You're only the patient—what's it got to do with you?

Jacqueline Worthington

The need for communication

It is easier for patients to accept the situation if their doctors are good communicators, which many are not. But it has to be said that even when careful and detailed explanations are offered, the confusion and anxiety associated with being in hospital makes it difficult for women to take in what they are told.

The midwife and doctors did try to explain what was going on and seemed quite sympathetic. But I wasn't really able to absorb what was happening and what might happen and just kept saying things like 'Do I have to have a Caesarean?'

Janet O'Toole

Doctors have to decide how far to go in outlining their anxieties about what might happen. If they pull their punches to soften the impact of the news they might later be accused of concealing the risks; if they are totally frank they could be accused of terrorizing a patient into compliance. Nobody wins in these circumstances, and it would be in everyone's interests for women to embark on pregnancy with a clearer and more realistic appreciation of all the potential risks (see Chapter 8).

In the worst cases, complications arise so quickly—and often unexpectedly—that there is no time for explanations. It is not all that rare for a happily pregnant woman who is feeling well and looking forward to a joyful delivery at full term to be plucked straight from an antenatal clinic into hospital, be dosed immediately with various powerful drugs and be delivered within hours of a premature baby which is taken away to fight for its life in intensive care.

If, as sometimes happens, such complications set in very early in the second half of pregnancy, the unfortunate mother may be confronted without warning with the horrific information that she must be delivered without delay to save her own life but that delivery will almost certainly kill the baby who is now moving so happily within her. This is a tragedy from which few women emerge without permanent psychological scarring.

My first baby was delivered stillborn at 24 weeks, 11 years ago. I know that this was necessary to save my life, but I have never got over the emotional consequences.

I started to feel unwell with abdominal cramps at around 22 weeks. My doctor poked around a bit and said everything seemed OK—but he didn't take my blood pressure. A couple of days later I was in agony, and this time he took my blood pressure. Hiding his shock at how high it was, he sent me straight to hospital.

But by the next day I had blood clotting problems and was showing signs of kidney failure. The doctors came to the conclusion that they couldn't save the situation and I was told that the only way of curing my problems and saving my life was to remove the baby.

So the next day they gave me the equivalent of a late abortion, but it didn't work, so they had to go in manually and literally rip the baby out of me. That was terrible! But even worse was the fact that, although they offered to show me my baby, it wasn't for long enough. I was still not totally *compos mentis* and not bright enough to say 'Leave the baby with me'. I feel I have never been able to mourn that baby properly—and that is something no one can ever put right.

Although I appeared to recover fairly well, every now and then the birth and its aftermath came back to haunt me—and still does after all these years. I thought that if I talked through what happened enough times the problem would gradually disappear—but it hasn't.

My immediate reaction was to throw myself back into work. It took about a year to decide to give motherhood another go. And this time I did get a live baby—even though she was born as early as 26 weeks.

Although I had no signs of pre-eclampsia this time, apparently the placenta was not functioning well and I threatened to go into premature labour at 23 weeks. I was kept in hospital, but eventually went into full labour at 26 weeks. My daughter Dawn, who weighed 710 g (1.6 lb), was the second smallest survivor the hospital had ever had.

I can't say it hasn't helped me to have Dawn—but it hasn't helped the mourning problem. Dawn has made my life more complete, but you can't replace one child with another.

June Jones

Allocating blame

It is common for pregnant women to blame themselves when things go wrong, but with pre-eclampsia such guilt is futile because there is no evidence that anything an individual woman does has any bearing on whether or not she falls victim to the disease.

Another common reaction, particularly in serious cases, is to blame doctors and midwives for failing to recognize early warning signs. Sadly, this accusation is sometimes justified, but it is important to understand that even if the warning signs *had* been noticed the outcome might not have been any different. Once pre-eclampsia has embarked on its destructive course it can rarely if ever be turned back, only neutralized by early delivery. Early diagnosis can help to prevent complications, but it cannot normalize the pregnancy.

CAN PRE-ECLAMPSIA BE PREVENTED?

Various claims have been made and various techniques tried over the years to prevent pre-eclampsia. However, because these have been geared to suppressing one or more of the outward signs of the disease, rather than the disease itself, they have not stood the test of time.

Diuretics

Diuretics, which abolish fluid retention by forcing the kidneys to excrete more water, were very popular 'preventive' agents about 30 years ago, when doctors thought that all oedema in pregnancy was an early warning of pre-eclampsia. But it soon became clear that the treatment made no impact on the incidence of pre-eclampsia. Moreover, it was recognized that diuretics, like all drugs, had side-effects, some of them dangerous. Nowadays, they are reserved for treating severe complications of fluid retention, such as pulmonary oedema.

Salt restriction

Salt restriction also enjoyed a vogue as a preventive technique—salt has been implicated in raising the blood pressure as well as causing fluid retention. But when the effects of salt restriction in pregnancy were tested in a large trial in 1958, it was found to be positively *harmful!* Women in the salt-restricted group not only had more 'toxaemia' than the controls, they were also more likely to lose their babies. The problem appears to be that the kidneys need a good supply of salt to work efficiently. If there is too little salt and the kidneys are under strain for other reasons—as they are with pre-eclampsia—they have fewer reserves and fail more readily. These days salt restriction has died out in most places, although it persists in some corners of the globe.

Control of blood pressure

Control of blood pressure has been seen as another way of preventing pre-eclampsia. For at least the last three decades it has been argued that even a moderately raised blood pressure could be causing 'damage' in some hidden and silent way, and that this explained the increased risk of pre-eclampsia for women with chronic hypertension. It seemed logical to assume that if the hypertension could be controlled then the extra risk of pre-eclampsia would disappear. The same argument was extended to the hypertension of early pre-eclampsia: surely, enthusiasts claimed, the hypertension was contributing to the progress of the disease and good control of blood pressure would halt it or at least slow it down. However, this theory has not been borne out by scientific studies and, although the issue remains controversial, doctors these days tend to reserve drugs for situations where the hypertension is bad enough to pose the risk of stroke.

Weight gain

Weight gain has been another target for so-called prevention. It is now known that the excess weight gain associated with pre-eclampsia is caused by fluid retention and so is not under the mother's control, but 10–15 years ago, doctors believed that at least some of it was attributable to overeating. This theory was reinforced by studies of countries coping with war-time food shortages, which appeared to show an associated decline in the incidence of pre-eclampsia. So it seemed that women brought pre-eclampsia upon themselves by greed. And from here it was a simple step to introduce diet restriction as a preventive measure. Women could be weighed regularly to make sure they weren't gaining too much, and those who developed pre-eclampsia could be chastised for not sticking to their diets.

There was—and is—little logic to this viewpoint. Moreover, scientists now know how important an ample, well-balanced diet is to the health of pregnant women and their babies, and that a poor diet may increase the risk of pre-eclampsia.

The *good* news is that scientists are starting to have some idea of which components of the diet are most important in the genesis of pre-eclampsia. Calcium appears to be beneficial, although it is not clear why, and so do the essential fatty acids found in oily fish, which have direct effects on blood platelets. We take a more detailed look at the evidence in Chapter 6 (p. 140).

'Low dose aspirin'

At present the most promising preventive technique of all is the administration of daily doses of aspirin to at-risk women. Aspirin also has beneficial effects on the platelets in pre-eclampsia, and these effects can be achieved with tiny doses—no more than one-fifth of an ordinary tablet taken just once a day.

Chapter 7 looks more closely at the preventive possibilities of aspirin, but meanwhile we must point out that the use of aspirin in pregnancy is still experimental, and no-one should take it except under strict medical supervision.

WHAT HAPPENS NEXT TIME?

Women who have suffered severe pre-eclampsia look forward to their next pregnancy with painfully mixed feelings. Those whose babies have died may be thrilled to be pregnant again but terrified that history will repeat itself; while those whose babies survived worry about who will hold the fort at home if they have to spend a long time in hospital again.

Couples in these situations need detailed and reliable information to help them cope, but they don't always get it. Sometimes (although rarely these days) doctors duck the issue by advising against further pregnancies—a harsh and devastating verdict that is scarcely ever justified. More commonly—but equally misleadingly —doctors tell their patients that 'it hardly ever happens a second time'.

In my next pregnancy I did not receive any special care and was told 'It shouldn't happen again.' But it did—and this time I suffered headaches and saw flashing lights, which did not happen the first time. It took about two weeks after the birth before my blood pressure even began to go down. I have my blood pressure checked regularly now, and have been told that

my problems in pregnancy could be a warning of blood pressure trouble
to come in middle age.

Jacqueline O'Hara

In fact, women who have suffered severe pre-eclampsia in a first
pregnancy have a 1 in 20 chance of succumbing to severe disease in
their next pregnancy; and their risk of mild pre-eclampsia is more
than three times higher than for those women whose first pregnancies were uncomplicated by any pre-eclampsia.

The risk of recurrence is increased by other predisposing factors,
such as kidney disease or chronic hypertension (see p. 88). For this
reason, women who have had pre-eclampsia should have a full medical check-up before they conceive again to make sure there are no
such hidden problems. The check-up should include an ultrasound
scan of the kidneys, measurement of kidney function, and a reassess-
ment of the blood pressure.

After one recurrence of pre-eclampsia, a woman is even *more* prone
to recurrence in a subsequent pregnancy, and with each further
recurrence the risk for the next pregnancy is multiplied. For women
who have suffered three serious attacks, the risks are so high that
they might well be advised to call it a day.

It is a good idea for affected women to discuss the next pregnancy
with their doctors well in advance. Although the outlook is good
for most women, there is no reason for complacency because it is
impossible to predict who will be unlucky. Only when the next
baby is safely in its mother's arms can anyone afford to relax.

A woman at risk of recurrence should be offered an individually-
tailored antenatal care plan, including frequent assessment by
specialists who understand the complexities of the disease. Unfortunately, few hospitals have the facilities to provide such a service,
although many individual consultants do their best under less than
ideal conditions. This is another argument for the provision of
specialist centres in each region (see Chapter 7).

Victims of pre-eclampsia often ask how long they should wait
before becoming pregnant again—a particularly sensitive issue if
the first baby has died. There is no standard answer to this question.
In general it is advisable to leave at least 6 months between one
birth—successful or otherwise—and the next conception, but after
that it is up to the couple themselves. There is no particular medical
advantage in waiting longer than 6 months, but there may be

sound *psychological* reasons for taking long enough to enter the next pregnancy in a resilient and optimistic frame of mind.

Some women worry about whether they should take the contraceptive pill in future, as it is known to exacerbate blood pressure problems. However, the Pill is unsuitable only if you suffer from chronic hypertension, in which case the progestogen-only or 'mini' pill is safer, although slightly less reliable as a contraceptive.

HOW TO HELP YOURSELF

If it were possible to prevent pre-eclampsia by making simple changes in your lifestyle, the disease would not be a problem and there would be no need for this book. However, the fact that you can't do this doesn't mean you can't help yourself at all and, in fact, there are a number of useful protective measures you can take either in a first pregnancy or after a previous experience of pre-eclampsia.

Diet

A good, balanced diet gives a good start: but it is misleading to suggest, as some advisers do, that this alone will guarantee protection from pre-eclampsia. It can't—but it will help.

Rest

Rest sounds logical, but is overrated. Living in the fast lane is never a good idea in pregnancy, but there is no need to wrap yourself in cotton wool for 9 months. Just do what you can easily cope with.

Antenatal care

Most important is close collaboration with the professionals who are providing your antenatal care. The dull routines you go through at each visit may seem pointless, but they offer the best available protection against the worst ravages of pre-eclampsia.

Always make sure your obstetrician is aware of your personal history of pre-eclampsia and any additional risk factors you have for the disease (see p. 88); and don't be afraid to speak up if you think the proposed interval between visits is too long. Our advice is that after 24 weeks at the latest the intervals between checks should not be longer than 2 weeks. If the first attack of pre-eclampsia was severe, then in your next pregnancy you should be offered weekly checks for at least 4 weeks before the stage when disaster struck last time.

Remember that the experts are not all that expert and few of those looking after you will be familiar with all the different complications of pre-eclampsia. For your part you should *never* skip an antenatal check—particularly after 20 weeks—however well you feel and however blooming you look. Remember that pre-eclampsia causes no symptoms until it reaches a late and dangerous stage.

There is no harm in keeping an eye on your own readings and making sure the appropriate steps are taken when necessary. If your blood pressure goes up suddenly you should be offered more frequent monitoring, in case it is the first sign of pre-eclampsia.

A urine test should be carried out—and the result recorded in your notes—at each visit. If ever there is protein (+ or more) in your urine, further tests are essential. The protein level should be rechecked in a clean (midstream) urine sample, which should then be checked for infection—sometimes a benign cause of mild proteinuria. A further recheck of all the readings is essential within the next week. If protein in the urine is combined with a raised blood pressure then you should be admitted to hospital, however well you feel and however inconvenient it seems.

Swelling on its own is not a cause for concern, but if it appears suddenly and affects your face as well as hands, feet and ankles then it may be significant. A sudden increase in weight gain to more than 1 kg (2.2 lb) per week is rarely normal and should lead to more thorough and regular checks—at least once a week.

Headaches are common in pregnancy and not necessarily significant. But a severe headache associated with vomiting and/or abdominal pain is a potentially sinister development, which should be checked out at once, preferably in hospital. You will need to stay in for at least a day and night to enable doctors to assess the stability of your blood pressure, if it is raised, and analyse a 24-hour urine collection if there is any suggestion of proteinuria. Blood tests to measure your platelet count and assess your liver and kidney function are needed to exclude more serious pre-eclamptic disturbances.

Some women would prefer to play a more active role in antenatal care by taking their own blood pressure and testing their own urine at home. This is a safe option only in very close liaison with a doctor and/or midwife, so that worrying readings can be double-checked without delay. It may well be a useful system for the future, although only a few centres are trying it out.

6 · In search of a cause

In the last two chapters we have made it clear that the main problems bedevilling the doctors who deal with pre-eclampsia are ignorance of the fundamental cause of the disease and uncertainty over precisely how it develops. If these were known, doctors would be able to develop accurate predictive and diagnostic tests and ultimately find reliable ways of treating and/or preventing the disease. Pinpointing the cause of pre-eclampsia—a quest currently occupying teams of research workers all over the world—is far from easy. It is clear from what *is* known that there is no simple cause-and-effect relationship as with, say, an infectious illness and the organism responsible for causing it. Like heart disease and cancer, pre-eclampsia is a multilayered condition, and the illness itself is only the final event in a sequence of disturbances, each of which may have more than one cause.

Current knowledge of pre-eclampsia is rather like an incomplete jigsaw, with parts of the picture clearly defined but important pieces missing. The known landmarks in the evolution of the disease include:

1. *Poor placentation.* In normal pregnancy, specialized embryonic cells, known collectively as the trophoblast, break down the walls of the uterine spiral arteries enabling them to dilate to many times their normal size (see p. 26). This adaptation, which is complete by the end of the first half of pregnancy, enables the arteries to carry a progressively increasing blood flow to the placenta in the second half of pregnancy. In pre-eclampsia the transformation of the spiral arteries is incomplete and they remain narrower than they should be.

2. *Placental ischaemia.* There comes a point in the second half of pregnancy when the supply of blood through the incompletely adapted spiral arteries fails to meet the increasing demands made by the placenta, which becomes *ischaemic* (short of blood) as a result. A vicious cycle is created because the ischaemia triggers off a further problem of *acute atherosis*, in which the spiral arteries become par-

tially blocked by fatty and other deposits, so aggravating the ischaemia.

3. *Fetal illness.* Babies affected by pre-eclampsia may show signs first of intrauterine growth retardation, caused by shortage of food, and later of oxygen starvation, both of which are consistent with an inadequate blood supply to the placenta.

4. *Maternal illness.* Mothers affected by pre-eclampsia first exhibit a range of symptomless clinical signs, including high blood pressure, proteinuria, dramatic swelling, and disturbances in blood clotting and liver function. The condition invariably gets worse until the baby is delivered, and can culminate in severe, even life-threatening, complications such as eclampsia (convulsions), cerebral haemorrhage, kidney failure, widespread clotting (DIC), oedema of the lungs, and liver damage.

5. *Effects of delivery.* The progress of the disease can be interrupted at any stage by delivery of the baby and placenta, which invariably leads to complete recovery unless irreversible damage has occurred.

Poor placentation gives rise to placental ischaemia, which in turn causes at first symptomless disturbances and finally overt and serious illness in mother and/or baby, unless interrupted by early delivery.

Other facts about pre-eclampsia have emerged from studies of affected women. It is known, for example, that the condition runs in families and is most common in first pregnancies; that women who have suffered in a first pregnancy are more likely to have pre-eclampsia in second or later pregnancies than those whose first pregnancies were normal; that certain factors peculiar to the pregnancy —such as multiple birth—and certain pre-existing medical problems—such as chronic hypertension—increase the risk of pre-eclampsia.

In summary, then, doctors know more or less *what* happens in pre-eclampsia and even *to whom* it is most likely to happen. But they don't know *why* and *how* it happens, so the picture is necessarily incomplete. What interferes with the crucial adaptation of the spiral arteries? Does the problem lie with the mother, the fetus or both? Why are first pregnancies particularly affected? How does placental ischaemia cause illness in the mother? Why are its manifestations so variable from woman to woman? Why does pre-eclampsia sometimes affect the mother but not her baby—and vice versa? Why is the progress of the disease sometimes sluggish, sometimes fast and furious? Why do some women never get it again while others suffer equally severely in pregnancy after pregnancy?

There is no shortage of theories to fill these gaps in the pre-eclampsia picture. An enormous number of environmental and other factors have at one time or another been credited with causing or influencing pre-eclampsia (see Chapter 2), ranging from external infection to internal toxins (hence 'toxaemia'); from too much food to too little food; from poverty to affluence; from the colour of a woman's eyes to—yes—the weather! Many of these have been disproved or considered unworthy of serious investigation.

Below, we describe and evaluate the most important current theories about pre-eclampsia. No one research team has as yet developed a unified hypothesis that covers the whole spectrum of the condition, from its placental origins to its most serious effects. Most have focused only on one part of the incomplete picture. So the ideas put forward are not mutually exclusive: indeed, there may well be some truth in all of them. Each may prove to be a more or less important link in the chain of understanding that will eventually solve the mystery of pre-eclampsia.

We start at the very top of the chain of events that unfold in pre-eclampsia, and look at why some women are more likely than others to develop the disease.

THE GENETIC THEORY

It is established beyond doubt that pre-eclampsia runs in families and that women whose sisters and/or mothers have suffered in their pregnancies are at much greater risk of the condition than women with no family history of the disease.

A major US study followed the sisters and daughters of a group of women who had suffered eclampsia and found that as many as 37 per cent of the sisters and 26 per cent of the daughters developed pre-eclampsia or eclampsia in their own first pregnancies. In comparison, the incidence for the daughters-in-law of affected women was only 6 per cent. These statistics suggest that pre-eclampsia is, at least in part, an inherited condition, passed directly from mothers to their daughters. However, no-one has yet identified a gene or genes that can be said to be responsible for causing pre-eclampsia.

A research team from Edinburgh University is currently working on the hypothesis that pre-eclampsia is a 'recessively-inherited' genetic condition. To clarify what that means we need to digress into a brief explanation of genetics.

The nucleus of each cell in our body contains 23 pairs of chromosomes—one of each pair is inherited from our fathers and the other from our mothers. Each chromosome is a string of many thousands of genes, each of which provides a blueprint for some individual function of our bodies by making one specific protein. When a gene is defective or faulty (and this can happen by chance or through inheritance), it makes a faulty protein that may, in turn, lead to malfunction of a particular organ. Like chromosomes, genes are paired, one of each pair inherited from the mother and the other from the father.

There is a huge degree of genetic variability among normal people, which accounts for many natural differences in body traits such as height, colouring, even blood pressure. Moreover, these genetic differences lead to marked variations in the way individuals respond to environmental challenges, including those that produce disease. Looked at in this way it is possible to describe every known disease as a result of interaction between a given individual's genetic make-up and the environment. In certain diseases, however, the genetic component is so overwhelming that it expresses itself regardless of other factors: these are known as 'genetic disorders'.

There are various categories of genetic illness and the group we are concerned with here are the simple or *mendelian* genetic disorders, which are determined primarily by a single defective gene, passed on by one or both parents to their children. The pattern of inheritance of such a disease may be *dominant*, meaning that a single defective gene, inherited from one parent, is sufficient to cause the disease even though the other gene in the pair is normal, or it may be *recessive*, meaning that the disease can occur only if *both* parents pass on the relevant defective gene. One such recessively-inherited disorder is cystic fibrosis, for which the responsible gene has recently been identified. There are many scientists who feel that pre-eclampsia is inherited in the same way, but their work has been hampered so far by failure to locate and identify the responsible gene.

The Edinburgh University researchers are studying a number

of families, in each of which there is a mother who has suffered pre-eclampsia and two daughters, only one of whom has been affected. They are hoping to localize the pre-eclampsia gene to a particular chromosome and ultimately to identify the gene itself and delineate its role in the human body. However, they are only likely to succeed if they are right in assuming that the disease is recessively inherited. If it follows a different pattern of inheritance, or if genetics is only one factor in its causation, then the picture is likely to be obscured.

The researchers themselves acknowledge that the gene is expressed fully only in a first pregnancy. So pregnancy itself must have an effect that somehow modifies the gene's expression in second or subsequent pregnancies. But the recessive theory doesn't explain, for example, why a minority of women suffer pre-eclampsia for the first time in a second or later pregnancy; or why recurrent pre-eclampsia is particularly likely after a change of partner.

Other researchers in this field believe that these quirks can be accounted for only by recognizing that the *baby's* genes, as well as those of its mother, have a role to play in the development of pre-eclampsia. Their theory is that the condition develops only if the baby, as well as the mother, has two copies of the relevant defective gene. They also believe that the predisposition to pre-eclampsia can be modified not just by a previous pregnancy but by other factors, including diet and drugs, particularly aspirin.

At this stage it seems unlikely that the genetic theory will be able to explain each and every case of pre-eclampsia, although it may well explain why some women are susceptible to the disease in their first pregnancies.

We know that the earliest detected event in the development of pre-eclampsia is failure of trophoblast cells to dilate the spiral arteries supplying the placenta. So if pre-eclampsia is a genetic disorder it must be mediated through some mechanism controlling either the 'invasiveness' of the trophoblast (which will depend on the baby's genes) or the receptivity of the maternal tissue (determined by the mother's genes)—or both.

The genetic theory cannot itself account for the low recurrence rate of pre-eclampsia, although this can be explained in other ways. For example, it may be that a first pregnancy physically alters the structure of the arterial blood vessels within the uterus in such a way that they never contract back to their original shape and so are much easier for trophoblast cells to dilate in subsequent pregnancies. But probably the most promising explanation for how the genetic inheritance is expressed and why it is expressed most strongly in first pregnancies is provided by the next theory.

THE IMMUNE THEORY

As we explained in Chapter 3 (p. 25), pregnancy is something of a biological paradox. How is it that although the immune system invariably recognizes transplanted organs as 'foreign' and makes strenuous efforts to 'reject' them, a human embryo, which is half foreign on account of its paternal genetic inheritance, is not only accepted but welcomed and nurtured? There are three possibilities:

(i) the embryo may be 'special' in the sense that it does not display its foreignness;

(ii) the uterus may be a privileged site, which is not affected by normal immune responses;

(iii) the mother's immune responses may be modified somehow during pregnancy to ensure the survival of the baby until full term.

So far no-one has been able to resolve this paradox by explaining the immunological basis of normal pregnancy, but scientists at the John Radcliffe Hospital in Oxford are working on the third hypothesis; they are aiming to prove that the immune adaptations of normal pregnancy go slightly wrong in pre-eclampsia so that the mother mounts a weak rejection response against the placenta as it becomes established in the first half of pregnancy. This rejection is not strong enough to cause total failure of the pregnancy but it can make the womb lining sufficiently hostile to the invading trophoblast to hinder the crucial adaptation of the spiral arteries.

The same process could be at work in some cases of recurrent miscarriage; but whereas with pre-eclampsia the immune response is weak enough to allow some degree of placentation, with miscarriage the rejection is so vigorous that placentation fails completely.

The immune theory of pre-eclampsia could explain its low rate of recurrence except after a change of partner. A first pregnancy would effectively 'desensitize' the immune system to the presence of the foreign genes, so they would not be treated in such a hostile fashion in subsequent pregnancies. However, a pregnancy conceived with a new partner, passing on a different set of foreign genes, would be threatened to the same degree as the first. The trouble is that the theory is as yet unproven, and will probably remain so until the immune responses of normal pregnancy are fully understood. So far it has been established that the innermost lining of the pregnant uterus—the decidua—is packed with immune cells that differ from those found elsewhere in the body and whose precise function is as yet uncertain. It is also known that the cells of the trophoblast lack all the usual signals of 'foreignness', properly known as HLA antigens. These antigens, which are inherited, play a major role in determining the success or failure of any organ transplant, and the fact that trophoblast cells lack these signals indicates that normal pregnancy (or 'nature's transplant') succeeds, at least in part, because the fetus is able to conceal its foreign identity behind its trophoblastic shell. However, there is no evidence so far that this pattern is in any way disturbed in pre-eclamptic pregnancies.

If proved, the immune theory of pre-eclampsia could be enormously beneficial; once the nature of the immune response were known it might one day prove possible to simulate the protective effects of a first pregnancy by desensitizing a woman's uterus to her partner's sperm before conception. But that is a development for the twenty-first century!

Of course, the immune theory is not essential for explaining how pre-eclampsia develops. Another possibility is that some women have less well-formed uterine blood vessels than others, with a reduced ability to dilate in response to the extraordinary demands of pregnancy. As the blood vessels never contract back to their original size after pregnancy and would therefore be easier to dilate in second and subsequent pregnancies, this would still be consistent with the known preponderance of pre-eclampsia in first pregnancies.

THE PLACENTAL ISCHAEMIA THEORY

The main defect of placentation in pre-eclampsia was first described in 1972 by a group of British and Belgian researchers. They examined small samples taken from the placental beds of pre-eclamptic patients at Caesarean section and found that only the decidual ends of the spiral arteries were dilated, while the sections running through the muscle of the uterus were unchanged. This finding has since been confirmed, and more recently it has been shown that in pre-eclampsia up to half of the 150-or-so spiral arteries that feed the placenta are completely unchanged. In other words, some of the arteries are not dilated at all, while the rest are only partly dilated. This means that the arteries are incapable of carrying the high volume of blood the placenta needs in the second half of pregnancy; as a result the placenta becomes ischaemic. This has been proved by postdelivery examination of pre-eclamptic placentas, which often show gross evidence of ischaemia, including infarcts—areas of tissue that have died owing to lack of blood.

The link between this placental ischaemia and the pre-eclamptic illness in the mother has now been established by animal experiments. Scientists have managed to induce the symptoms of pre-eclampsia in pregnant animals by artificially blocking the blood supply to their placentas. The most recent research has been carried out by researchers from Sydney, Australia, who have so far induced the symptoms of pre-eclampsia in half a dozen pregnant baboons by tying off one of the two uterine arteries early in the second half of pregnancy, so halving the blood supply to the placenta. The results were sudden and dramatic: in each case, the baboon's blood pressure rose, followed by a fall in the platelet count and the appearance of proteinuria. Although none of the baboons died, one needed an emergency delivery to prevent what appeared to be an imminent eclamptic fit. As with the human version of the illness, all the pre-eclamptic signs returned to normal after delivery.

However, a vital link in causal chain is still missing: ischaemia in itself is not enough to cause all the many and varied features of pre-eclampsia, and most experts believe that the illness is caused by a substance, or substances, produced by the ischaemic placenta and released into the mother's body. This resembles the old theory that the pre-eclamptic woman was overwhelmed by toxins circulating in her blood—a theory that gave the disease its early title 'toxaemia'. We shall refer to the mystery substance as 'factor X'.

THE FREE RADICAL THEORY

What is 'factor X'—and how does it operate? Most promising among the candidates currently being considered are *free radicals*— short-lived, unstable, highly-reactive, and potentially destructive by-products of oxygen metabolism.

Free radicals are characterized by the presence of one or more unpaired electrons. Electrons are small particles of electricity that spin in one particular direction and are extremely reactive unless paired with other electrons with an opposite spin. Free radicals are generated when the bonding between an established electron pair is broken. So desperate are the 'free' electrons to find another mate that they can seriously damage the structure of the cell by breaking up other, previously stable, electron pairs. This can set in motion a violent chain reaction in which disruption moves like a wave through part of a cell, leaving behind a trail of damage.

Free radicals are produced naturally in our bodies as by-products of the burning or *oxidation* of food to release energy. Some free radicals are thought to be useful: for example, they help to kill bacteria and parasites. But free radicals are so potentially destructive that they need to be strictly controlled. Our bodies keep them in check by producing substances that 'scavenge' or neutralize them; these include a number of enzymes and vitamins with *antioxidant* properties, particularly vitamins C and E. Unless this natural protective mechanism works well, free radicals can run riot in the cells, damaging their membranes and sometimes even killing them or altering their genetic codes in such a way as to cause mutation.

Such harmful free radical reactions have been implicated in the causation of many degenerative diseases, including cancer, heart disease, and arthritis. Some scientists believe that the very process of ageing itself is caused in large part by a progressive reduction in natural protection against free radical reactions, leading to increased tissue damage.

Free radicals are known to be produced after tissues have become short of oxygen because of ischaemia: indeed it is possible that much of the damage associated with heart disease is caused not by the ischaemia itself but by the consequent over-production of free radicals. So it is logical to assume that they might be produced in excess in ischaemic placentas, and there is some evidence that this is so. Free radicals tend to home in on the unsaturated fatty acids present in all cells, converting them to rancid products known as *lipid peroxides*. Low levels of lipid peroxidation are essential to many normal cellular processes; but uncontrolled peroxidation can damage cell membranes. Not only that but lipid peroxides formed at one site can be transported in the circulation to cause further damage at more distant sites.

A major overview of studies on lipid peroxidation in pregnancy, carried out by researchers from the US universities of Vermont and California, found several indications that blood levels of lipid peroxides are higher in pre-eclampsia than in normal pregnancy. It has been suggested that lipid peroxidation may play a role in causing the disease. Animal studies provide evidence to support this hypothesis. For example, a US experiment carried out in 1959 showed that rats fed a diet of peroxidized (rancid) fat and kept short of the antioxidant vitamin E in early pregnancy developed a number of changes resembling human pre-eclampsia in the latter stages of their pregnancies.

The US researchers suggest that placental ischaemia intensifies the release of placental lipid peroxides into the mother's circulation, with harmful results.

Whatever the identity of 'factor X', it is likely that it operates by damaging the innermost lining of the mother's blood vessels. This inner coating—the *endothelium*—is made up of a continuous sheet of flattened *endothelial cells*, which have a number of important, protective functions. These functions are known to be disturbed in pre-eclampsia.

THE ENDOTHELIAL CELL DAMAGE THEORY

This theory, put forward by the same US researchers who outlined the free radical peroxidation theory above, goes one step further and explains how the consequent damage to the endothelial cells lining the blood vessels might be a direct cause of the maternal illness in pre-eclampsia.

First, there is good evidence that endothelial cell injury is a common feature of pre-eclampsia. The most consistent structural abnormality associated with the disorder is glomerular endotheliosis —swelling and increased permeability of the endothelial cells lining the capillaries of the kidneys' tiny filtering units, known as glomeruli (see p. 35).

The biochemical evidence of endothelial cell injury is even stronger: two factors known to be released from injured endothelial cells—fibronectin and factor VIII-related antigen—are increased in the blood of pre-eclamptic women.

Endothelial cells have many important functions: they hold blood and its contents within the vessels, allowing two-way transport of nutrients and waste products in a precisely regulated manner; they help to stop the platelets from gathering together (aggregating) to form unnecessary clots, and they protect the blood vessels from a number of agents that tend to constrict them.

When endothelial cells are injured, all these functions are disturbed, partly by the injury itself and partly by the natural defensive mechanisms brought into play to limit blood loss from damaged vessels. The platelets become overactive and the blood more prone to clotting, while the blood vessels close down in spasm. In addition, the vessels may become more permeable or 'leaky' than usual.

These known effects of endothelial cell injury fit with the clinical features of pre-eclampsia: the leakage of fluid from blood vessels into the tissues; the leakage of valuable proteins from the bloodstream into the urine; the clotting disturbances; and the excessive constriction of the blood vessels, which ultimately causes high blood pressure.

Damaged endothelium disturbs the platelets, and vice versa: overactive platelets can also disturb the endothelium. So the endothelial cell damage theory is closely tied to theories that implicate the platelets.

THE PLATELET THEORY

Increased platelet activity, ultimately leading to clotting disturbances, is a well-known feature of pre-eclampsia. As more research is completed it seems increasingly likely that the platelets are involved at a very early stage.

A team of US scientists from the Wayne State University in Detroit recently established that women who go on to develop pre-eclampsia show signs of enhanced reactivity of the platelets as early as the end of the first trimester of pregnancy. More specifically, they demonstrated that the platelets showed an exaggerated response to a particular chemical agent that is known to activate platelets and constrict blood vessels.

If this finding is borne out by other, larger, studies it could provide the basis for a test to predict the onset of pre-eclampsia as early as 12–14 weeks. Equally importantly, it would indicate that the platelets play a more fundamental role in the development of pre-eclampsia than has been assumed so far; and this would explain why the disease appears to be modifiable by antiplatelet agents, particularly low-dose aspirin.

What causes this enhanced platelet activity at such an early stage of pregnancy, before the placenta has had a chance to become ischaemic and release 'factor X', is not clear, but it could be connected with a chemical imbalance in the placenta, which is known to occur in pre-eclamptic pregnancies.

A recent study by a scientist from Michigan State University in the United States found that in normal pregnancy the placenta produces equivalent amounts of *thromboxane*—a hormone-like substance that tends to activate platelets, constrict blood vessels, and stimulate uterine activity—and *prostacyclin*, a related substance with the opposite effects. However, while the pre-eclamptic placenta produces three times as much thromboxane as the normal placenta, it produces less than half as much prostacyclin—in consequence the ratio of thromboxane to prostacyclin in pre-eclamptic pregnancies is 7:1. So the effects of thromboxane predominate in pre-eclamptic pregnancies, while those of prostacyclin are diminished, which helps to explain the increased constriction of the blood vessels, enhanced platelet activity, and reduced placental blood flow, which are characteristic of the condition. These effects would tend to accelerate as the pregnancy progresses, as activated platelets produce more thromboxane, thereby exacerbating the existing imbalance. The damage would not necessarily be restricted to the placental circulation—there is evidence that the thromboxane and prostacyclin produced by the placenta are secreted into both the maternal and fetal circulations. The thromboxane/prostacyclin imbalance could also reduce the blood flow from the placenta to the fetus because thromboxane constricts the umbilical artery.

A more recent study carried out by US pharmacologists at the Vanderbilt University, Nashville, Tennessee, found that the production rate of thromboxane in pre-eclampsia was highly correlated with the severity of the illness. As aspirin suppresses thromboxane production from platelets, this is another justification for its use in preventing pre-eclampsia. The authors of this study suggest that it should also be evaluated as a potential treatment for diagnosed pre-eclampsia, when it might limit the severity of the disease.

DIETARY THEORIES

It has been believed for many years that dietary factors play a role in the development of pre-eclampsia, but at what point they enter the chain of events is not clear.

Although some extravagant claims have been made for the importance of diet in pre-eclampsia, it seems most likely that an individual's dietary status serves to modify or amplify other factors responsible for the illness, rather than being a direct cause itself.

One of the most important studies to date on the link between diet and pre-eclampsia was carried out in Britain just before the outbreak of the Second World War, when the People's League of Health appointed a special committee to consider the influence of nutrition in pregnancy on maternal and infant health.

In a pretrial exercise, nearly 1000 pregnant women recorded everything they had eaten for a week and the records were then analysed for signs of deficiency. The vitamins and minerals most commonly found wanting—particularly calcium, iron, and vitamins A, B1, and C—were incorporated into supplements to be used in the trial proper.

More than 5000 pregnant women attending the antenatal clinics of 10 London hospitals were enrolled in the trial; all were less than 24 weeks pregnant and in good health. The women were divided into two groups, one receiving a daily dose of the nutritional supplements and the other left untreated. The incidence of pre-eclampsia was only one of the outcomes measured in the trial, but the results were startling—pre-eclampsia affected 7.4 per cent of the first-time mothers in the untreated group but only 5.4 per cent of those in the treated group.

Interestingly, although the trial organizers expected that those who had taken the supplements for longest would have the lowest incidence of pre-eclampsia, the best results were obtained by those who took them for only 16–20 weeks. This suggests that dietary status cannot be a primary cause of the disease.

Another interesting point about this trial is that part of the daily supplement taken by the treated group was given in the form of halibut liver oil, a rich source of vitamins A and D. Very recently scientists have begun to suggest that fish oils, including cod and halibut liver oils, may play an independent role in modifying the course of pre-eclampsia. Fish oils are rich in a particular type of fatty acid that is present in large amounts in the human retina and brain. For this reason alone fish oil may be of great importance in the diet of pregnant women and supplementation with fish oil may be particularly appropriate for women at risk of pre-eclampsia. This is because the fatty acids contained in the oil inhibit the body's production of thromboxane which, as explained above, activates platelets and constricts the blood vessels, so aggravating the circulatory problems of pre-eclampsia.

Future studies may show that fish oil supplementation is a useful alternative to low-dose aspirin for preventing pre-eclampsia. But these are early days and fish oil supplements are not yet recommended during pregnancy, particularly as some sources are also rich in vitamin A, which is suspected of causing birth defects when taken in excessive amounts.

Another component of the supplement used in the pre-war dietary study that has begun to assume independent significance is calcium. A recent study carried out in the Ecuadorian Andes, where people have a low calcium intake, looked at the effects of calcium supplementation in 56 healthy first-time mothers, all of whom showed a rise in blood pressure at 28–32 weeks of pregnancy and were therefore considered at risk of pre-eclampsia. Half of the women were treated with a daily calcium supplement until delivery and the other half were given *placebo* (dummy) tablets. Only 14 per cent of women in the calcium group went on to develop pre-eclampsia but 71 per cent of those taking placebo tablets fell victim to the disease. Further studies are now under way to substantiate these important implications.

Much more grandiose claims for the effects of diet have been made by Thomas H. Brewer MD, author of *Metabolic toxaemia of late pregnancy: a disease of malnutrition* (Keats Publishing Inc., 1982). Dr Brewer makes the following statements:

1. Pre-eclampsia (which he calls 'metabolic toxaemia of late pregnancy') is not primarily a placental disorder but a disease of malnutrition, causing liver damage, which somehow (Brewer is rather vague over this) gives rise to the classic sign of pre-eclampsia.

2. Pre-eclampsia has been virtually eliminated in certain areas of the world among women who receive good nutrition and good prenatal care. This is simply not true—neither is there any discernible class gradient in the incidence of pre-eclampsia.

3. Pre-eclampsia is entirely preventable by a good, well-balanced diet in pregnancy, with emphasis on high-quality proteins, vegetables, and fruit—an unsubstantiated claim.

Brewer's claims are based on his own experience. In 1963 he began a research project at the county prenatal clinic at Richmond, California, with the aim of getting every patient to adopt a high-protein diet, including 1.25 litres (2 pints) of milk, two eggs, and two portions of fish or lean meat per day. In the book, first published in 1966, he says that in the first 235 of those patients whose hospital records he studied there was not a single case of (pre-eclampsia). In an afterword to the 1982 edition he updates these statistics and says that in more than 7000 pregnancies managed with his 'methodology' there was not a single case of eclampsia and no maternal death.

Brewer's ideas have been embraced wholeheartedly by the Pre-eclampsia Society (PETS), a British charity, which recommends 'the Brewer diet' to women seeking information on how to prevent pre-eclampsia. But Brewer undoubtedly claims more for the importance of diet than is fair. He has not attempted to validate his theory scientifically with a controlled clinical trial—in which a group of women would be randomly assigned either to treatment with his diet or to no dietary advice; and his attempts to explain how malnutrition causes pre-eclampsia are unconvincing. Neither does Brewer's theory accord with what is known about pre-eclampsia. If it were indeed a disease of malnutrition then it could be expected to occur most often in the lower socio-economic groups, which does not happen. And malnutrition cannot explain the predominance of pre-eclampsia in first pregnancies.

SUMMARY

In summary, none of these theories, proven or not, can provide a complete explanation for pre-eclampsia. It may even be that pre-eclampsia is not a single illness but the final common manifestation of several different pregnancy disturbances, each with its own starting point.

We must also point out that none of the theories is sufficiently established to justify indiscriminate intervention. We *do not* advise pregnant women to dose themselves with fish oil, calcium, vitamin E or aspirin. When the experts are uncertain, consumers are unlikely to get it right, and misuse of some of these preparations could do more harm than good.

7 · Towards a better future

'Those who cannot remember the past are doomed to repeat it,' warned the American poet and philosopher George Santayana. This is a sad truth about the approach of doctors and midwives to the problems of pre-eclampsia and eclampsia; bitter lessons have been learned over the years and then forgotten, perpetuating much unnecessary suffering. Again and again the worst, most tragic complications arise when too little is done too late, usually despite the presence of clear warning signs. Over the past 40 years a clear record of this neglect has accumulated in the Department of Health's triennial *Reports on Confidential Enquiries into Maternal Deaths in England and Wales*. Since 1952, the first year covered by these reports, pre-eclampsia and eclampsia have consistently been one of the four main causes of maternal death, and were *the* main cause in 1982–4, just as they were in 1952–4.

Great progress has been made in the interim, and pregnancy and childbirth have become safer in many ways. But while the *number* of deaths from pre-eclampsia/eclampsia has declined from 200 in 1952–4 to 25 in 1985–7, their relative importance as a *proportion* of total maternal deaths has not.

The most consistent and important problem highlighted by these reports is substandard care—in other words neglect. We need to look at this problem in some detail since it underlines an urgent need for change.

THE NEED FOR BETTER CARE

In the three years 1952–4, 200 women died of pre-eclampsia or eclampsia in England and Wales. Death was judged by the assessors of the *Confidential Enquiries* to have been 'avoidable' in 52 per cent of these cases, the most frequent avoidable factor being 'faulty antenatal care'.

In the next report, for 1955–7, when 171 women died of pre-eclampsia/eclampsia, the assessors were more stringent in their criticism, pointing out that hypertensive disease had retained its 'unenviable position' as the most important cause of maternal death. 'Faulty antenatal care,' they added:

is by far the most serious and most frequent avoidable factor and the faults recorded in this series could be regarded by most doctors as inexcusable in these days.

By 1958–60, the number of deaths from hypertensive disease had fallen to 118, but 56 per cent of these were still judged to be avoidable. Only in 1961–3 did the proportion of avoidable deaths fall to below half, but only just, at 49 per cent.

In 1967–9, when there were 53 deaths, 66 per cent of them avoidable, the assessors began for the first time to comment on the role of specialist obstetricians. Consultant responsibility for avoidable deaths included:

. . . a poor standard of antenatal care . . . failure to take action when signs of toxaemia were first observed, delay in admitting a patient to hospital and further delay in taking action when worsening signs and symptoms presented.

From 1973 onwards, two trends were evident, one good, one bad. The good trend was the continuing, if slow, reduction in the number of deaths; the bad one was an apparent increase in the proportion of avoidable deaths, most of them involving substandard care by consultants. The 1973–5 report pointed out:

Greater vigilance is necessary in the early detection and treatment of hypertensive disease in pregnancy . . . high risk patients were seen too seldom, patients with signs of pre-eclampsia were not admitted promptly and, in particular, procedures, such as caesarean section, were too often delegated to inexperienced junior staff . . . The reports of deaths of patients with pre-eclampsia make a sad story of neglect.

The problem was not—and is not—confined to this country. US obstetrician Lester Hibbard, reporting on maternal deaths in Los Angeles, wrote in 1974:

Physician error contributes greatly to acute toxemia deaths. Prominent among these errors are . . . underestimation of the virulence of the toxemic process; . . . reluctance to apply the only definitive therapy yet devised— termination of pregnancy.

Of course it is easy to be wise after such tragic events. While clinical staff are always rushing from case to case, making instant decisions, the armchair specialist can use what is jestingly known as the 'retrospectoscope' to see what should have been done. Nevertheless, the judgements that have emerged from the *Confidential Enquiries* demand to be taken seriously because they have been made not by bureaucrats or intellectuals, but by practising doctors who know the pressures their colleagues are under but *still* believe better care should have been given.

In 1979–81 the authors of the *Confidential Enquiries* stuck their necks out and suggested action to solve the continuing problem of substandard care. 'Severe disease,' they acknowledged:

is sufficiently rare to make it difficult for every obstetric unit to maintain continuous expertise in its management . . . We therefore suggest that in each region it would be valuable to have one or more teams with special expertise . . . Early detection and expert management of severe hypertensive diseases of pregnancy would help to bring about the improvement in maternal mortality from these disorders which has been so disappointingly absent in the past decade.

In 1982–4, when consultants were implicated in 16 out of the 18 deaths in which care was considered substandard, the assessors pointed to the continuing need for 'regional teams with special expertise'.

So, although there has been impressive progress in treating the disease over the last 40 years it remains, as always, a disease of neglect. This is not to say that all specialists are neglectful—far from it; indeed where care has been substandard, the lapses have been occasional rather than consistent. Nevertheless, these lapses amount to a tragic waste.

The case for Regional Centres

Although a solution to the problem of neglect has been proposed, it has not been embraced wholeheartedly by the specialists themselves. Regional centres specializing in pre-eclampsia/eclampsia are being set up, but only in some parts of the country, and where they *do* exist, some obstetricians are reluctant to use them because of the loss of face involved in referring patients elsewhere.

We believe this attitude is out of date. Pre-eclampsia is such a complex, variable disease that few obstetricians have the time to learn enough about it from the handful of very severe cases they see each year. Also, while the management of severe pre-eclampsia demands continuity of care extending over days and sometimes weeks, obstetric units are organized around the needs of labouring mothers, whose problems last for 24 hours at most. Almost all of them find it difficult to maintain a high level of continuous care for longer than this.

The development of super-specialist regional centres for pre-eclampsia will be boosted by new programmes of training, which make it easier for obstetricians to specialize in particular areas of interest. As more of these 'subspecialists' are trained, it will be a natural development to centralize their skills in special units, but even then it will still be up to individual obstetricians to decide whether to refer their patients to these units. True progress will only come when it is generally recognized that the level of care currently on offer is just not good enough.

The ultimate goal of everyone concerned with pre-eclampsia must be to eradicate the disease completely. Such a feat would revolutionize maternity care, removing a key justification for the 'medicalization of childbirth' so resented by many women. Without the spectre of pre-eclampsia there would be no need for the regular weigh-ins, blood pressure checks, and urine tests that form the cornerstone of the antenatal programme; and the total number of antenatal visits needed could be halved at least. Inductions, Caesarean sections, and other interventions would be reduced and more and more women could reclaim their pregnancies and their birth experiences for themselves. But the key to this happy future is more knowledge.

THE NEED FOR MORE RESEARCH

It is possible for a disease to be conquered before it is properly understood: one example is smallpox, where vaccination was used long before the smallpox virus was identified. But it is usually necessary to know your enemy inside out before a strategy can be devised to ward it off. So more research is needed—and particularly answers to the following questions:

- Why is pre-eclampsia primarily a disease of first pregnancies, and why are most women well protected in later pregnancies but others not at all?

- What exactly interferes with placentation in pre-eclamptic pregnancies?

- What is the link between the sick placenta and the maternal illness?

- Why is the maternal illness so variable? Could it be that there is more than one disease process involved?

- Why are some babies severely affected by the placental problem and others not at all?

- What causes eclamptic fits and why do only a minority of severely affected women suffer them?

- What genetic and environmental factors are involved?

These questions need to be answered, not in broad outline but in exact detail, so that every landmark in the evolution of pre-eclampsia is understood from every possible angle. Only when it is known for certain what causes the initial fault and how one link in the chain of events gives rise to another will it be possible to devise ways of blocking what now seems a relentlessly progressive disease process.

Research workers face three main obstacles to furthering these goals:

1. They can't expect to work out what goes wrong in pre-eclampsia until they understand what is supposed to happen normally. Many doctors and scientists around the world are working towards a fuller comprehension of the processes of normal pregnancy; this knowledge will be relevant not only to pre-eclampsia but also to the understanding and treatment of infertility, recurrent miscarriage, and preterm labour—and even to the development of better contraceptive methods.

2. Facilities for studying pre-eclampsia as it develops in humans are very limited. Scientists can study placental cells after delivery and deduce what went wrong in retrospect, but they have no direct access to working placentas or to cells from the mother's kidney, liver, and brain—all of which might be affected by pre-eclampsia.

3. Obstetrics is a low priority area for research—both in terms of scientific interest and grant allocation. Charities like Action Research and Birthright support research related to pre-eclampsia, but both are small. Big organizations, like the Medical Research Council and the Wellcome Trust, have more money, but scientists researching the problem of pre-eclampsia must compete for grants with many others covering the whole field of medicine and human biology.

Funding

Most, if not all, research on pre-eclampsia is carried out in hospital obstetrics departments. For historical reasons these have been slow in developing their research capabilities—not just for pre-eclampsia but for all complications of pregnancy—and so often lose out in open competition for funds. To become competitive these departments need to attract the best scientists but, in a classic Catch 22 situation, the best scientists won't come because obstetrics is an area of low prestige and poor funding.

For many conditions, including cancer, heart disease, and kidney disease, to name but a few, dedicated charities have been established with a prime aim of raising funds for research; many of these have been highly successful. This has not yet happened for pre-eclampsia, although the condition must have touched the lives of at least one million families in the UK. This, too, could be an important direction for the future.

The need for a 'model' of pre-eclampsia

Progress in research will be improved if an animal 'model' can be found for pre-eclampsia—in other words if scientists can study the disease as it evolves in experimental animals more closely than is possible with humans. Workers in Australia and the United States have found that they can induce something that looks like pre-eclampsia in pregnant baboons or rhesus monkeys by a surgical procedure that starves animals' placentas of blood (see p. 135). Now, with this technique, the link between placental ischaemia and the clinical signs of pre-eclampsia can be examined more directly. However, this can only help to explain the later stages of the disease, not the fundamental placental disorder.

Cellular research

Meanwhile, other workers are learning more about the basic processes of placentation—how the placental cells interact with their maternal host cells in the decidual lining of the womb. This work has been made possible by the availability of placental tissue after abortion—now a sad but inevitable part of life in most Western countries. The inner lining of the womb during placentation is a social gathering of many different types of cells, some in conflict, others engaged in various co-operative activities. Current research should eventually enable scientists to make sense of this society of cells, which is the frontier between mother and baby and a key to understanding the function and health of the placenta. Such studies should lead to an understanding of what happens to these cells in the very early stages of pre-eclampsia, but to find out *why* it happens scientists need to identify the gene or genes that make some women susceptible to pre-eclampsia in pregnancy (see p. 130).

The human genome project

The last decade or so has seen massive advances in our understanding of genes, and 1990 saw the launch of the Human Genome Project, a massive and costly world-wide effort to catalogue the structure and map the location of every single gene in the human body, storing the information on an international computer database. When the catalogue is complete it will include the culprit(s) responsible for pre-eclampsia hidden somewhere among the 100 000 genes we are estimated to carry on our chromosomes. But identifying the pre-eclampsia gene will reveal only its structure, not its function. Further work will be needed to find out what the gene's role is in the normal workings of the human body and how it is perverted in pre-eclampsia. To make matters even more complicated, scientists may need to look for more than just a maternal genetic factor in pre-eclampsia, because it may well be that, although the mother needs to have a genetic susceptibility to pre-eclampsia, the disease is only sparked off in the presence of particular *fetal* genes, as inherited from the father.

Scientists are a long way from reaching a full understanding of the many processes involved in pre-eclampsia, but this should not stultify progress in the detection and management of the disease. The would-be parents of today cannot wait for scientists to solve these weighty problems before they start their families; and there is much that can be done now to improve their prospects.

THE NEED FOR BETTER TESTS

Although pre-eclampsia is common, 9 out of 10 pregnant women do not get it. If these fortunate people could be identified at the start of their pregnancies, their antenatal care could be simplified considerably. Conversely, if those who were destined to suffer the problem could be identified in advance they could not only be offered more intensive screening at more frequent intervals but could also be targeted for specific measures designed to prevent or ameliorate pre-eclampsia.

Ultimately, it may prove possible to pick out the women who will go on to develop pre-eclampsia by demonstrating that they (and maybe also their partners) carry the relevant genes. Such tests could be carried out before couples start their families so that affected pregnancies could be monitored and treated from the very start. However, it could be many years before such tests become available, and meanwhile scientists are exploring other ways of replacing the crude and unsatisfactory techniques currently used to assess whether individual women are at low or high risk of pre-eclampsia (see p. 95).

There are three possible bases for predictive or diagnostic tests:

1. *Platelet activity*: a recent study by workers in Detroit (see p. 138) has indicated that abnormal platelet activity—a characteristic feature of pre-eclampsia—can be detected as early as the end of the first trimester in women who subsequently develop pre-eclampsia. If this finding is confirmed by larger studies, it could provide the basis for a remarkably early test.

2. *Endothelial damage*: many of the maternal problems in pre-eclampsia are thought to be caused by damage to the endothelial cells lining the blood vessels. Damaged endothelial cells release specific substances into the bloodstream (see p. 137) and blood levels of these substances are frequently raised before pre-eclampsia becomes evident. However, this is an imperfect way of predicting pre-eclampsia, as the endothelial cells can be affected by other unrelated disturbances in the mother's body. Endothelial cell damage is also probably a relatively late event in the pre-eclamptic process and is therefore unlikely to be detectable early enough to enable doctors to influence the course of the disease.

3. *'Factor X'*: if scientists knew the identity of the substance, or substances, released by the ischaemic placenta and causing the maternal illness, this could be measured in blood samples to give absolute proof that the disease was developing. This would revolutionize the accuracy of diagnosis

and, at a stroke, put an end to the endless and unproductive arguments about how to define the disease. Then, after two thousand years as a 'syndrome'—merely a collection of characteristic symptoms or signs— pre-eclampsia could be elevated to the status of a disease with its own unique features. The substances most likely to fit the 'factor X' bill are products of free radical activity (see p. 135), but much more work is needed before this can be confirmed.

THE NEED FOR PROGRESS ON PREVENTION

If the description we have given of the evolution of pre-eclampsia in Chapter 4 is correct, the development of actual illness in the mother is the last chapter in a much longer story. By the time the mother and her doctors are aware of the problem it is almost certainly too late to do anything but make the best of a difficult, irreversible, and unpredictable situation.

Any preventive measure that is going to work will need to be employed very early in pregnancy, long before the signs of the disorder appear. This again highlights the need for a good predictive test for the accurate identification of women likely to benefit from such treatment. Alternatively, it may prove possible to devise preventive measures that could be safely offered to *all* women before their first pregnancies. Doctors know that the best possible protection against pre-eclampsia is having been pregnant before. If they understood how pregnancy conferred this protective effect and could learn to simulate the effect before pregnancy then the incidence of pre-eclampsia could be reduced dramatically. This is the ultimate goal of research workers who believe that pre-eclampsia is triggered by overactivity of the immune system, leading to partial 'rejection' of the embryo by the mother (see p. 133). A logical concomitant of this theory is that pregnancy effectively 'desensitizes' this jumpy immune system so that pre-eclampsia is much less likely to occur in subsequent pregnancies. If this hypothesis is correct then it might prove possible in future to develop a form of desensitizing 'immunization', which could offer the same protection in advance of the first pregnancy.

Aspirin

Meanwhile, other possibilities offer more immediate hope of progress in preventing pre-eclampsia. Most promising is the use of small daily doses of aspirin—between one-quarter and one-fifth of a normal tablet—throughout pregnancy. So far, low-dose aspirin has been used only on an experimental basis, but the results of the first small trials show that it really *does* help to prevent the maternal illness. What is not yet certain is whether aspirin helps babies affected by pre-eclampsia; neither is it clear just how safe it is—for mothers and babies—to take aspirin in pregnancy; and this must be known before it can be wholeheartedly recommended for use in preventing pre-eclampsia.

One potential side-effect of aspirin is impaired blood clotting: low-dose aspirin appears to help prevent pre-eclampsia by 'damping down' overactive platelets, but as these specialized blood cells play a vital role in clotting activity, it is possible that aspirin could, in rare cases, lead to dangerous bleeding in either mother or baby. It is also possible that aspirin could have unforeseen effects on the later growth and development of the child. No-one has any reason to suspect or anticipate such an influence, but it must be ruled out before aspirin can be recommended.

Reassurance on both these points can come only from properly organized trials of the use of aspirin in high-risk pregnancies. Such trials have to be large to be really useful because uncommon side-effects might escape detection in a group of only 100 women, but would probably be picked up in a trial involving several thousand.

The current multinational CLASP trial (Collaborative Low-dose Aspirin Studies in Pregnancy), organized by the UK Medical Research Council, is expected to involve more than 9000 women from the UK and other countries. It is what is known as a 'randomized, double-blind, placebo-controlled trial'—the type most likely to yield accurate and credible results. Half the subjects are assigned by a random process to receive aspirin tablets and the other half are given identical-looking inactive pills (placebo). In each case neither the woman nor her doctor knows whether she is on active treatment or placebo—this is what is meant by 'double-blind'—so that the outcome cannot be influenced by expectation (the placebo effect). Only afterwards, when the outcomes of all the pregnancies are known, are the contents of the tablets revealed, allowing a comparison of the aspirin group with the placebo group.

If the incidence of severe pre-eclampsia is significantly reduced in the aspirin group then aspirin will have been shown to work—at least as far as the mothers are concerned. Doctors involved in the trial are hoping that it will be extended to include follow-up of all the children so that any long-term influences on their health can become apparent.

The scale of this trial is so large—it involves more than 100 hospitals in the UK alone—that it requires special organization to co-ordinate the world-wide activity. Twenty years ago the infra-structure for such endeavours did not exist and, as a result, the trials that were carried out were always too small to yield absolutely reliable information, which is why doctors cannot be certain of the advantages of many of the different treatments used in the management of pre-eclampsia, including anticonvulsant and anti-hypertensive drugs.

The need for rigorous testing

Any potential treatments developed in future, however miraculous and harmless they may appear, can only be recommended after they have been tested as rigorously as aspirin. The problem is that trials like these, although totally acceptable in most branches of medicine, are controversial in pregnancy because risks may be incurred not just by consenting adults but also by their unborn babies. The thalidomide tragedy, among others, has made pregnant women, doctors, and drug companies extremely nervous when it comes to testing drugs in pregnancy.

This is a very sensitive issue, requiring close co-operation between doctors and consumers. It is vital that new treatments should not be introduced until their safety and efficacy can be demonstrated in large trials; but progress will only be made if women are prepared to take part in such trials.

The use of fish oil supplements might be a case in point. The essential fatty acids in fish oil affect the platelets in a similar way to aspirin (see p. 140) and might be a useful alternative for preventing pre-eclampsia. Fish oil may sound safer—in the sense of being more natural—than aspirin, but it could pose a similar risk of haemorrhage, as well as causing other unforeseen side-effects of its own. Only a very large-scale trial could balance the potential benefits against the risks.

Another area of treatment that needs to be assessed in trials is the control and prevention of eclamptic fits, which is unsatisfactory, to say the least. It will undoubtedly be very difficult to carry out a trial in the middle of what is always an emergency situation, but most doctors agree that the nettle must be grasped. Before any such trial can be set up, information is urgently needed about the incidence of eclampsia and in what circumstances fits occur. Amazing though it may seem, no-one knows the scale of the problem. Most obstetricians see less than one case of eclampsia per year, so no-one has any kind of overview and experience of the problem is dispersed between almost a thousand UK specialists. There has never been any kind of national survey, although steps are now being taken to set one up. And no one knows the number of cases per year, to whom they occur, and whether they occur *despite* treatment or for lack of it.

We have covered many important issues in this chapter and thrown down a number of challenges for doctors and scientists. But what about mothers themselves: do they have a role to play? In our view, yes!

THE NEED FOR CONSUMER PRESSURE

The questionnaire survey carried out for this book (see Chapter 8) drew responses from hundreds of women, who clearly welcomed the chance to air their feelings and share their thoughts about their experiences of pre-eclampsia, and these must represent only the tip of what looks like a pretty large iceberg. Such women need a national body to provide a forum for their views and act as an effective pressure group on their behalf. Until recently, there has been only one such organization which, in our view, has taken a narrow line by espousing an unproven dietary theory.

However, in 1992 the authors of this book helped to found a new charity, Action on Pre-eclampsia (APEC), which aims to offer support and broad-based information to families affected by pre-eclampsia. APEC also aims to educate the public and health professionals about the condition, campaign for improved methods of detection and treatment, and raise funds for vitally needed research.

For more information about APEC, write with SAE to 61 Greenways, Abbots Langley, Herts, WD5 0EU, or call the Helpline on 0923 266778.

SUMMARY

In summary, then, although the future looks promising, the road is long and arduous. We believe the main priorities must be more research on all aspects of pre-eclampsia and all potential treatments; better organized, more specialized care; and a strong alliance between everyone whose lives are touched by the disease—doctors, midwives, and parents. These should hasten us towards the ultimate goal of eradicating pre-eclampsia entirely.

8 · How women cope with pre-eclampsia

So far we have dealt at great length on pre-eclampsia as a physical disease: how and why it develops, its complexity, its variability, its unseen perils, how it is understood by scientists and managed by doctors, current problems, and future solutions. What has been missing so far is any sense of how it *feels* to suffer pre-eclampsia. What is it like to be happily, confidently pregnant one day and seriously ill the next? How do women cope with their disappointed expectations of pregnancy and, in the worst cases, the loss of a longed-for child? What do they think of the care they receive? How are they affected in the long term?

We obtained answers to these questions through a questionnaire survey of women's experiences of pre-eclampsia, distributed with the help of several magazines and a national newspaper. The questionnaire, which attracted hundreds of respondents, was originally conceived as a means of gathering information for the case histories that appear in Chapters 4 and 5, but, although most of our respondents gave very clear accounts of the illness and its consequences, they wrote most lucidly—and movingly—about their thoughts and feelings.

The same themes recurred in questionnaire after questionnaire: the reluctance of women to anticipate anything but a perfectly normal pregnancy and delivery; the frustration and resentment they felt at being confined to hospital, often feeling perfectly well; confusion at doctors' failure to explain the nature of the illness and its possible outcomes; fear compounded by a sense of 'loss of control'; a perception of being 'cheated' of a normal experience; feelings of failure, guilt, and bitterness; depression and a lack of confidence in the future; a need to attach blame—to themselves or their doctors; terror that it would all happen again next time; a universal and unanswerable cry from the heart: 'Why did it happen to me?'

Any serious illness is liable to leave emotional as well as physical scars, but pre-eclampsia seems a particularly potent source of psychological trauma—it is not simply a horrible and dangerous disease but a perversion of a normal process, which is expected to have a happy outcome. The shock of such an unexpected setback, fuelled by inadequate preparation, is then compounded by the failure of at least some health professionals to explain what is going on and to involve their patients in discussions and decisions about their care and treatment. Several of our respondents reported that their experiences had caused them to lose their faith in doctors. This reaction was most common in women who had felt unwell and sensed that something was wrong but had their fears dismissed out of hand without proper investigation. Pre-eclampsia is the most common serious complication of pregnancy and the major justification for regular antenatal checks: but it is difficult to avoid the conclusion that some doctors and midwives are alarmingly complacent in their approach to potential victims.

The bitterest feelings were expressed by women who had lost their babies, in many cases after coming close to death themselves. Their sad stories exposed a number of weaknesses in an admittedly overstretched health service: inadequate support and counselling; lack of time or inclination to explain exactly what happened and why; insufficient discussion and reassurance about future pregnancies.

When we analysed the questionnaires it became clear that a number of changes were urgently needed in the way not just health professionals, but also women themselves, approach the problem of pre-eclampsia. Below we outline these needs, supporting our views with direct quotations from the questionnaires.

WOMEN SHOULD BE BETTER INFORMED

I am still amazed at the lack of information available. When I tell anyone about my experience of pre-eclampsia they are baffled because they have never heard of the condition—and that includes people with children.

Moira McGrory

Pre-eclampsia, in all its forms, affects one pregnant woman in 10, which adds up to more than 50 000 women every year. But for such a common—and such a dangerous—condition, it has an absurdly low profile.

Pregnant women are an easy target for health educators, because the vast majority attend antenatal clinics. The standard 'booking-in' visit to hospital around the end of the first trimester presents an obvious opportunity for midwives and doctors to draw attention to pre-eclampsia as the major justification for the regular checks that will punctuate the pregnancy from then on. However, as Jacqueline O'Hara pointed out, this opportunity is all too often missed:

I had never heard of the disease first time. Even after reading all the leaflets handed out at the booking-in clinic I was none the wiser. On the fateful morning I was admitted I had joked to my husband 'I don't know why I am going to this clinic—they never tell you anything different!' I did go, of course, luckily for me. But if I hadn't it might have been too late.

Parentcraft classes are another logical forum for education about pre-eclampsia but our impression is that these tend to focus on the aspects of pregnancy over which women are deemed to have some control—healthy eating, regular rest, exercise to alleviate minor discomforts, breathing techniques for labour, etc.—and to gloss over medical risks that seem to reduce women to the level of victims. This was highlighted by Gillian Samuel:

When I attended antenatal classes they just explained the good side of things and about perfect pregnancies. I now know it doesn't work that way.

Angela Paterson went further:

So much emphasis is put on 'natural childbirth' today (by the NCT, for example) that if things don't go smoothly the guilt felt is greater and a sense of failure persists. I was totally unprepared for anything other than a perfect, natural delivery.

Pre-eclampsia receives scant attention from the ever-burgeoning range of maternity handbooks. Gordon Bourne, an authority quoted by many pregnant women, devotes only three-and-a-half pages out of a total of nearly 600 to the subject in his classic guide, *Pregnancy* (Pan Books, 1984). Sheila Kitzinger, another respected childbirth 'guru', gives it just over one out of 350 pages in her book *Pregnancy and childbirth* (Michael Joseph, 1980). Most of the current handbooks tend to emphasize the positive, normal aspects of pregnancy and underplay the risks, thus fostering the potentially harmful delusion that women can control the outcome if only they look after themselves properly.

I have a general complaint that pregnancy books shy away from all problems for mothers and babies. Most books are very patronizing and take the line 'don't worry your little head about such matters' . . . But since things can and do go wrong, surely it is much better to be prepared than to pretend it is always a rosy experience.

Olivia Timbs

In some cases the information given about pre-eclampsia is misleading and downright inaccurate. For example, in a half-page section on pre-eclampsia in *Caring for your unborn child* (Thorsons, 1990), the medical journalist Roy Ridgway says: 'A mild case can be cured quite easily with bed rest and it won't affect the unborn baby . . .' In fact there is currently no effective 'cure' for pre-eclampsia except delivery and bed rest serves no useful purpose for mild cases.

This, and other handbooks, manage to convey the false impression that severe pre-eclampsia is preventable and therefore rare. This can only serve to convince victims that either they or their doctors must have been at fault for the disease to have progressed so far.

A charitable interpretation of the reluctance of childbirth educators to pay due attention to pre-eclampsia is they don't want to alarm women unnecessarily and encourage them to think of pregnancy as a form of illness and themselves as passive victims. But in evading the issue they are doing a great disservice to the many thousands of women every year who do become ill in pregnancy and who are, in most cases, entirely unprepared for the problems they encounter. Is it not time for the balance to be redressed?

Pregnant women should have the full facts of what could happen to them clearly and sensitively explained. We need to be fully informed if we are to detect any problems early, before they become serious. We should not be protected from vital information.

Sheila Creighton

It goes without saying that all the respondents to our questionnaire had suffered pre-eclampsia at least once, in most cases severely, and were therefore speaking with hindsight. Women who have gone through such a shattering experience naturally have an insatiable appetite for any information they can lay their hands on. But are women who are just embarking, full of happy hopes, on their first pregnancy prepared to listen to warnings? Quite possibly not.

One respondent, from Bristol said:

Personally I chose to ignore any information about complications in pregnancy because I didn't think it could happen to me.

Another, from Manchester, put it even more forcefully:

I was the type of person—aren't we all?—who thought 'I am a healthy person: my pregnancy will be flawless, the delivery will be natural—no epidural for me!' Consequently I skipped the pages of maternity books covering what can go wrong in pregnancy.

So there is a risk that helpful information will fall on deaf ears. Nevertheless, someone has to shatter the idealized image of pregnancy that makes women unreceptive to warnings in the first place.

So what information should pregnant women be offered about pre-eclampsia? We think it should cover the following points:

- The nature and incidence of the disease;

- Who is most at risk;

- The importance of antenatal checks for detecting the first signs;

- Symptoms requiring urgent investigation;

- Current methods of management and the need for monitoring in hospital;

- Prospects for prevention and cure.

A brief factual leaflet could be produced to cover these points. More detailed information on risks, treatment options, and prospects for future pregnancies should be reserved for women who subsequently develop the disease.

PROFESSIONALS SHOULD BE MORE VIGILANT

At 34 weeks I had swollen ankles, high blood pressure, and a trace of protein in my urine. The community midwife noted these symptoms but took no action. I stayed at home most of the following week, feeling generally ill and tired and noting that my legs and ankles became more swollen. I was admitted as an emergency from a hospital antenatal class to the labour ward only because at the end of the class I had asked the midwife to check me over. I had read most of the current popular books on pregnancy and saw very little on pre-eclampsia—other than the implication that it is picked up in routine antenatal checks. I went to all these checks and still slipped through the system.

Anon.

Such anecdotes cropped up with alarming frequency in our questionnaires, indicating that doctors and midwives may be slow to diagnose pre-eclampsia even when the classic triad of symptoms—raised blood pressure, protein in the urine, and oedema—is present.

Raised blood pressure alone is not necessarily an indication for hospital admission, although it obviously calls for more frequent monitoring. But the appearance of protein in the urine, a sign that kidney damage has occurred, signals the onset of severe pre-eclampsia, which should always be managed in hospital because the condition of mother and/or baby can deteriorate rapidly.

The appearance of such symptoms as abdominal pain and vomiting, visual disturbances, and headache marks a late and dangerous stage of the disease. But they can be mistaken for common minor discomforts of pregnancy like indigestion.

I first realized something was wrong at 23 weeks. I had put on a lot of weight and had albumen (protein) in my urine and oedema of the hands and feet. Later I had severe pains in my stomach area. I went to my GP and told him that I feared I was suffering from pre-eclampsia. He told me that I was worrying about nothing. The pain became much worse, usually at night. I would roll around the floor or bed in agony. The local GP, when called each time, diagnosed indigestion, prescribed the usual remedies and gave me morphine injections. On Christmas Eve, the locum GP refused to treat me and sent me to hospital. They gave me another morphine injection and sent me home. One week later my husband took me to hospital again, frightened by the responsibility of caring for me. My blood pressure was 180/130 and I was kept in for two-and-a-half weeks before delivery. My baby died three days later.

Rudi Reeves

The tale told by Margaret Garrard was even more harrowing:

At about 33 weeks I was waking up in the morning with very puffy eyes, swollen fingers, and feet, which would go down during the day. I was due to go to the hospital in a few days, so thought I would mention it then. At this stage I didn't think anything was drastically wrong. (One evening) I was very sick and had a terrible headache. My husband 'phoned our GP, who prescribed paracetamol. My husband and I went to bed that night at 10.00 pm, hoping that the headache would subside. We both went to sleep. I had a fit at about 11.30 and swallowed my tongue and was turning blue. My husband put me in the recovery position and pulled my tongue forward to get me breathing again. He then 'phoned for an ambulance. I had another fit in the ambulance *en route* to Orpington Hospital, where I had another fit in the casualty department. In the early hours of the morning Jonathan was born by Caesarean section . . . I was very lucky that my husband, being a policeman, first-aid trained, and able to stay calm in an emergency, was there. I am very grateful to him for saving my life.

It is not just GPs and community midwives who are at fault when it comes to diagnosis and appropriate treatment. Women in the apparent safety of a hospital bed can also be neglected as Barbara Prescott revealed:

After delivery I complained of headache and vomited several times . . . No concern was shown. I asked for an aspirin and was refused and was left alone until the doctor came—more than an hour and a half after delivery. I complained again of headache—which by then was very severe—but no blood pressure was taken. My head began shaking from side to side involuntarily and the next thing I knew I was in a darkened room, feeling drowsy. No-one explained, but I had suffered an eclamptic fit. I was in that room for five days. By the time they brought my son I had no feeling for him. I couldn't grasp that he was my baby.

Doctors and midwives need to be more consistently vigilant in their screening for pre-eclampsia. Women with raised blood pressure and/or excessive weight gain (1 kg per week or more) should be monitored more frequently than usual; if the blood pressure is raised and then protein (+ or more) appears in the urine, hospital admission should be arranged the same day; and women who complain of feeling ill should always be given the benefit of the doubt and checked over as a matter of urgency: if other signs of pre-eclampsia are present they should be admitted to hospital by flying squad (see p. 101).

For their part, pregnant women need to learn to take more responsibility for themselves and to err on the safe side with symptoms (see Chapter 5, p. 125).

DOCTORS NEED TO TALK TO PATIENTS

The responses to our questionnaire suggest that it is not uncommon for doctors to admit women with pre-eclampsia to hospital and keep them there, sometimes for weeks at a time, without providing an adequate explanation of what is wrong, what is being done and why, and what may happen in future.

There may well be good reasons why doctors find it difficult to discuss pre-eclampsia with their patients: they don't have much time; the prognosis is nearly always uncertain, particularly when the baby is very premature; their scope for treatment is very limited; their patients are often ignorant, frightened, and desperate for reassurance. Nevertheless, the following extracts from responses to our questionnaire make it quite clear that for some women not knowing what was going on was the most harrowing aspect of their ordeal;

I was admitted straight from my last check at the GP's, just before 40 weeks, with very high blood pressure—it had been slightly raised from 36 weeks. He just said he would prefer me to be 'started off'. I was horrified: I didn't know why I was being treated so urgently, but my questions were sidestepped . . . I became so ill—I believe I had to be resuscitated at one point—that I had to have an emergency Caesarean, after which I didn't recover consciousness for 4 days. The gravity of my condition and even its name were never mentioned. I returned for my postnatal check and went away feeling that I was at fault, that I was a bad person to have caused so much trouble, and felt somehow bereaved as if something undefinable had been taken away with no explanation.

Chris Cox

Prior to delivery I was not given any information about what was happening to me so I was very confused—I simply couldn't understand what was happening. I was never consulted or informed about plans, so when I was taken to the labour ward for induction I thought they had made a mistake —got the wrong person. The anaesthetist arrived to give the epidural and I remember sending him away saying he had come to the wrong room— I still had 6 weeks to go. I just wish someone had taken the time to tell me exactly what was happening and why.

Ruth Vincent

I wondered why no one was volunteering any information and why they were so obsessed with my headaches and 'flashing lights'. I was very frightened but received no reassurance. I was left alone for long periods. I was scared of dying or my baby dying. I feel I was treated badly in the sense that I was told nothing by anyone. I was treated like a child throughout.

Sandra Jones

Some staff who *did* manage to convey the seriousness of the condition presented the information in an insensitive, even brutal manner.

On my birthday my husband asked a hospital doctor if he could take me out for a while. The reply was 'Well, you can if you want to, but your wife could go into a fit and die.' Obviously, we never went!

Angela Duxbury

No information about the illness was given to me. One evening a nurse woke me to give me a sleeping pill. I laughed at the stupidity of it. She told me: 'You are a stupid girl—your baby is dying inside you and all you can do is laugh!' Fourteen years later I can still recall the exact words!

Christine Tomlinson

Surely it is not too much to expect a doctor to sit down with a patient and explain what is wrong, what is being done to help, and what may happen in future? In some cases this will mean preparing women for the possible death of a baby, but what is the point of keeping them in the dark? As June Jones pointed out:

There is nothing more terrifying than not knowing what is happening, why it is happening and what the outcome may be.

We are not talking here about the adequacy or otherwise of medical treatment, but about patient care in its fullest sense. One respondent from Midlothian said:

I knew they were taking good care of me 'medically', just not 'personally'. I asked lots of questions and became very frustrated at not getting straight answers. I even became quite paranoid during ward rounds when 'they' would discuss me in the corridor before coming to my bed.

Christine Tomlinson picked up on the same point:

I think I had good, i.e. safe, treatment. But the rounds were like being visited by a member of the Royal Family. I should have liked more information, more contact.

It is the persistence of the traditional ward round, with teams of doctors gathered at the foot of a patient's bed, discussing her in the third person in terms she cannot understand, that enables doctors to maintain a distant, uncommunicative relationship with their patients; in our view this practice should be abolished. It is perfectly feasible for obstetricians and their teams to discuss the technical details of individual cases in private before the ward round begins, so that all dialogue at the bedside involves the woman and any members of her family who wish to be present. This more personal approach should give women the courage they need to ask the questions that most concern them. It is to be hoped that doctors in turn will find the courage to deal fully, honestly, and sensitively with these questions.

Good lines of communication are equally, if not more, important after delivery, when the illness is over, particularly if the baby died or the woman was dangerously ill herself. Women need to know what happened and why in order to come to terms with the situation and put it behind them. And the question on most women's lips is 'Will it happen again next time'. Doctors should be very careful about how they answer this question, and a full discussion on the next pregnancy may be best postponed until the 6-week postnatal check, when the woman is likely to have made a full physical recovery.

Some women enjoy perfectly normal subsequent pregnancies after suffering severe pre-eclampsia or even eclampsia; others endure successive problems; some have one or more normal pregnancies followed by a recurrence of pre-eclampsia (see p. 89). Doctors can quote statistics on the likelihood of recurrence but they can never be sure what will happen in any individual case. Pre-eclampsia is, as we have already pointed out, a disease of exceptions rather than rules.

Some doctors make a practice of telling women who have suffered in a first pregnancy that it hardly ever happens twice. This is simply not true, and several of our respondents were shocked and dismayed by the unexpected recurrence of a condition they had been led to believe was a one-off. A respondent from South Wales wrote:

After suffering severe pre-eclampsia in my first pregnancy I received no special care in my next pregnancy even though I had been told I would be carefully watched. The hospital disclaimed all knowledge of what had been said previously and I was told that I could not have pre-eclampsia in a second pregnancy and that I was over-anxious. When I started to feel ill again quite early in the pregnancy my GP felt I was over-anxious and would not take my blood pressure because he thought you couldn't have pre-eclampsia before 28 weeks. Eventually I felt so bad that I refused to go home at an antenatal appointment until I was allowed to see the consultant. He admitted me to see a neurologist because of headaches and visual disturbances. Once the neurologist confirmed that these were due to high blood pressure I was kept in hospital from then on—28 weeks—until delivery eight weeks later.

At the very least, any woman who has suffered pre-eclampsia in one pregnancy should be offered more frequent monitoring the next time around.

WOMEN SHOULD ACCEPT THEY ARE NOT IN CONTROL

I was admitted to hospital at 27½ weeks with high blood pressure and protein in the urine and delivered 4 days later by Caesarean. My main feeling on being admitted was shock. I was kept fully informed but I just couldn't believe it was happening to me. I was upset at first, but then I thought 'mind over matter' and tried to be very positive. I felt determined they wouldn't have to deliver my baby. Then I was just more and more dismayed when my blood pressure was so erratic.

Caroline Sharp

Many women, particularly those who have thought and read a lot about pregnancy, are prey to a delusion that the outcome of the pregnancy rests entirely in their hands; that if they don't drink or smoke, if they eat a healthy diet, get plenty of rest, and do their breathing and stretching exercises they will enjoy a perfect, healthy pregnancy and an easy delivery without need of medical intervention.

Of course, there are connections between lifestyle and the outcome of pregnancy. It is well known, for example, that smoking tends to restrict fetal growth while very heavy drinking can cause both physical and mental damage to an unborn baby. But in the present state of knowledge there is no proven connection between lifestyle and pre-eclampsia, and therefore no indication that you can cause it by neglect or prevent it by taking extra care.

It was clear from the responses to our questionnaire that many women who had been responsible enough to establish healthy lifestyles before and during pregnancy felt outraged by their failure to influence the outcome. 'Why me?' echoed through questionnaire after questionnaire.

I feel very angry at times. For example, I don't smoke and didn't drink through pregnancy, looked after myself and this happened. Then I see girls who have really abused themselves have one healthy baby after another. How can doctors explain that?

Anon.

They can't, of course; for there is no blueprint to ensure a trouble-free pregnancy and a healthy baby. You can do your best to weight the odds in your favour, but to a large extent every pregnancy remains a lottery.

For some women the sudden realization that they are not in charge of their pregnancies is one of the hardest things to bear about pre-eclampsia. Margaret Barnes wrote feelingly:

I have the sort of job and lifestyle where I feel I am 'in control'—and I found being hospitalized, with every decision out of my hands, quite terrifying. It took me about five years to recover mentally from not being 'in control' during those traumatic months. I do not regard pregnancy as an enviable state—I did not enjoy any aspect of mine; it has made me very negative about the 'magic' of being pregnant that some women describe.

To argue that women cannot control their bodies in pregnancy might appear to be a counsel of despair, but in fact the converse is true. It is women who believe their fate *is* in their own hands who suffer most when things go wrong.

Take the vexed question of blood pressure, for example. Women who believe they are in control are convinced they are pushing it up with their own anxiety and can bring it down by conscious relaxation. This puts them under almost intolerable pressure when being monitored in hospital, as Tracy Hall pointed out:

Every time I had my blood pressure taken I used to panic, knowing I had to try and relax to bring it down. I am sure my readings would have been lower if I had been at home.

Of course, high blood pressure is only a sign of pre-eclampsia, not the problem itself, and no amount of relaxation can bring it down to normal levels. Nevertheless, some women focus on hypertension as the root cause of all their troubles.

I felt powerless and helpless, because there was nothing I could do to stabilize my blood pressure and go home.

Kay Roberts

Women who seek control are also setting themselves up for long-term feelings of guilt, failure, and inadequacy after pre-eclampsia, forever searching for something to blame themselves for.

I still blame myself. My body let me and my son down. I don't really know what I did wrong, but it must have been *something*.

Alison Hoather

It is vital for such women to be reassured that they were not responsible for causing the disease and could not have done anything to prevent it.

DEPRESSED AND GRIEVING WOMEN NEED HELP

I experienced pre-eclampsia as long ago as 1957—it was then called pregnancy toxaemia—but the distress and heartbreak it caused us have never completely gone. My son was delivered by Caesarean section at 32 weeks. When I was told I would need an emergency Caesarean I was not a bit worried: it was Mothering Sunday and I remember thinking how wonderful it would be to become a mother on that day. When I came round from the anaesthetic I was told that I had to be very brave—our son had not survived. The next few days were an inescapable maze of shock, grief, and misery . . . I kept being told: 'Forget about it, you're young, you can have another baby'. I didn't want another baby, I wanted that baby. No-one suggested that we might want to see our little son. What actually happened to his little body we shall never know. I felt I would never be really happy again. I went on to give birth to two beautiful daughters, but I still think of my son every Mothering Sunday. I don't think the grieving ever stops.

Edna Benson

It is hard for any woman to come to terms with a pregnancy that culminates unexpectedly in a serious illness and a premature birth. But those who go through all the shock, fear, and anguish of the illness and emergency delivery only to lose their babies in the end endure the worse suffering. 'You never suffer anything worse than your child dying,' said a respondent from Potters Bar whose first baby died three days after a very premature delivery.

Losing a baby is particularly tragic for first-timers, who are also robbed of their anticipated status as mothers. They may have given up work, decorated the nursery, bought all the equipment, got to know other local mothers. Then suddenly the prospect of mother-hood is snatched away and they must somehow pick up the threads of their former lives again, although they feel forever changed. Meanwhile, physical reminders of their experiences like episiotomy stitches or Caesarean scars; swollen, aching breasts; and flabby tummies linger to prolong the torment.

Such women need sensitive handling and long-term counselling if they are not to succumb to depressive illness that might threaten their marriages as well as their future motherhood prospects.

I had a Caesarean at 28 weeks and my baby lived for only one hour. I recovered physically after about three months but I have never recovered mentally. I believe the whole situation contributed to the break-up of my marriage. The situation has also brought an end to another relationship as my boyfriend wanted children desperately but I could not face all the trauma and heartache.

Anon.

Thankfully, attitudes to bereavement have altered considerably since Edna Benson's day, when dead babies were quietly disposed of with-out contact with their mothers. These days it is normal practice for women to be given their babies to hold and cuddle and encouraged to hold funerals, all of which may help with mourning. However, some health professionals still seem to labour under the delusion that a dead baby is only a temporary set-back and that all will be well once the next pregnancy is under way.

When Joshua died on the third day, I just wanted to go home. The doctors and staff seemed unable to cope with the death. Even after the baby had died, I was asked to express milk for the other babies in the unit. My registrar, on hearing abut our baby, said: 'Never mind, you'll have another one next year.

Rudi Reeves

Of course, friends and relatives sometimes say the same sort of thing in a clumsy attempt to 'cheer up' a bereaved mother, as Jacci Fitch discovered.

My baby Hannah was delivered at 30 weeks but had stopped growing at 28 weeks. She died four days later. For a long time I couldn't hold anyone else's baby or talk about babies in general. I got married, had a baby and buried my baby all in the same year. People kept saying 'Oh you're young, you can try again'. That doesn't bring your baby back though: nothing can. It's something you can never get over—you just have to live with it.

Women like these need time to come to terms with their feelings, and counselling should extend beyond the hospital stay and the postnatal period, enabling them to work through their feelings and complete their mourning before they are ready to get on with their lives. Anger, usually directed against doctors, is often part of this grief and doctors should be prepared to keep discussing details of the illness, answering questions as honestly as possible, until their patients are ready to 'let go' of the experience.

Sometimes victims of severe pre-eclampsia suffer extreme psychological distress, even when their babies survive. Chris Cox was a case in point:

After the birth I had severe depression and spent most days alone at home clutching my baby, feeding him, loving him, and weeping. I told no-one and didn't go out much, feeling weak, and insecure. I collapsed into a dark and tormented mental confusion, well hidden from my family. My husband had a vasectomy and I grieved for the loss of my fertility, for the long years of confusion and misery ahead and for my own inability to have a baby properly. I felt like a genetic misfit.

For some women the illness casts a giant shadow over their relationship with the baby who 'caused' it. A respondent from Leicester suffered an eclamptic fit after giving birth to her first child in 1967 and was then sedated for three days. She recalled:

Because I did not have close contact with my baby for this time, 'bonding' was absent. It took more than three months to recover my fitness and I 'blamed' my daughter for taking away my good health. I had to seek psychiatric help in trying to bond our relationship. I could never feel close to her and often rejected her. It has had a long-lasting detrimental effect.

There is a sense in which women whose pregnancies went badly wrong are in mourning, too; they mourn the 'perfect pregnancy' and 'natural birth' they never got to enjoy, their belief in their power to control their own bodies, and their pride in their womanhood. Their difficult adjustment can be aggravated by the worry of caring for a premature baby, as Sheila Creighton discovered.

For a long time I think I was depressed, although I didn't realize it. I felt a failure and I found other people's reactions difficult to cope with: they didn't know whether to congratulate me on the premature birth of my daughter in case she died. Because she arrived so early I was totally unprepared for her both physically and emotionally. I had not attended any antenatal classes. The house was not ready for her. I didn't know how to cope with a tiny baby and felt terribly anxious. During the time she was in hospital and I had been discharged I felt very strange—I had a baby and yet I didn't feel she was mine. Other people didn't know how to react to my situation. I was tearful and confused.

Of course it is not just mothers who bear the emotional scars of pre-eclampsia. Fathers suffer too, often having faced the prospect of a double bereavement—wife and baby. But the fact that they are expected to be strong for their wives' may lead them to bury their own feelings. So it is vital that counselling be made available to the couple rather than the wife alone.

My husband suffered terribly. He was fully aware of the danger both I and our baby were in, whereas I was so drugged I was unaware of the dangers. He had to spend 2 days waiting to see if we would both pull through.

Mrs S. Vince

'My husband lost all his hair with the shock,' reported a respondent from Bristol, 'and it has never returned.'

When and whether to risk another pregnancy is a highly-charged issue for women who have suffered pre-eclampsia, particularly if the baby died. Some women cling to the prospect of pregnancy as a means of healing their grief.

Having lost my first baby, I desperately want to get pregnant again to prove to myself that it will be all right, that I am not fated for life.

Caroline Sharp

Others want to try again but are paralysed by fear.

After losing my first baby as a result of pre-eclampsia and the second because the pregnancy was ectopic, my husband and I have come close to nervous breakdown. We feel as if we shall never have children and our experiences have made us rather wary of trying again.

Elizabeth Winterton

Others take steps to rule out subsequent pregnancy:

I would have liked more children, but my husband had just as bad a time mentally, thinking he was going to lose his child and his wife and he decided to have a vasectomy to safeguard against further pregnancies.

Lynda Morrison

Women who do embark on a second pregnancy after suffering severe pre-eclampsia in the first need endless reassurance as well as careful monitoring in the next pregnancy.

I am now pregnant for the second time and throughout this pregnancy I have been unable to relax. I feel I am living on a tightrope and I won't feel back to normal until the baby is born safe and well.

Anon.

For some women, particularly those who have lost a first baby, the burden of pre-eclampsia cannot be lifted until they have experienced a normal pregnancy and held a full-term child in their arms. Even then, while the new baby may be a consolation and much loved in its own right, it can never replace the one that is lost. Doctors, midwives, health visitors, and other counsellors must understand this if they are to offer genuine support and understanding.

To end this chapter on an optimistic note, there is probably no new mother happier than one who experiences a normal pregnancy and delivery after a bad brush with pre-eclampsia. So we leave Angela Bird, a mother of five, to round things off:

My first pregnancy seemed like a nightmare for so long afterwards that it was six years before I plucked up enough courage to try again. But my second pregnancy was perfect and totally restored my confidence in pregnancy and in myself. The twins were born normally, five minutes apart, after a labour lasting five-and-a-half hours. I can still remember the exhilaration I felt that lasted for days afterwards. I'm so glad I found out what it was like to have a normal pregnancy and birth—there was no stopping me after that.

9 · Your questions answered

As the previous chapter suggests, many women are left confused and bewildered by their experience of pre-eclampsia, still living with such unanswered questions as: 'Why did it happen to me?' 'What did I do wrong?' 'Why did the pregnancy have to end?' 'Why did no one explain what was happening?' 'Can I be sure of a better experience next time?'

In this chapter we have attempted to answer these and other typical questions about pre-eclampsia as straightforwardly as possible. You will find very little new information here—it is mostly covered elsewhere in the book. But you might find the chapter helpful as a ready reference either before or after you read the main body of the text.

QUESTIONS AFTER DIAGNOSIS

Why has this happened to me?

No-one can say for sure: pre-eclampsia is a hereditary condition, but not in the purely genetic sense: there are well-documented cases of identical twin sisters with exactly the same genetic constitution, only one of whom suffered pre-eclampsia in her first pregnancy. It is presumed, therefore, that heredity decides whether or not a woman is susceptible to pre-eclampsia, but that the disease itself has to be 'triggered' by some extra—but so far unknown—environmental factor(s). However, many women who suffer pre-eclampsia have no family history of the condition, so even *this* explanation may be wrong (see p. 88).

What did I do wrong?

Nothing: there is no evidence that anything you do—or fail to do—in pregnancy has any bearing on whether you go on to develop pre-eclampsia, although personal or medical neglect might well enable preventable complications to develop (see Chapters 4 and 5).

If my doctor had picked up the warning signs sooner could the illness have been prevented?

No. At present doctors do not have the knowledge or the power to 'normalize' a pre-eclamptic pregnancy, however early the signs are picked up. Nevertheless, medical vigilance—including prompt diagnosis, close subsequent monitoring, and well-timed delivery— is vital for preventing dangerous complications of the disease; indeed it can make the difference between life and death for some babies —and even some mothers! (see Chapter 5).

Why do I have to stay in hospital when I can rest much more easily at home?

The purpose of admission is not to force you to rest but to enable your doctors to keep one step ahead of an unstable, unpredictable condition. Being in hospital is a form of insurance: during the worst sort of pre-eclamptic crisis, expert help is needed immediately and *any* delay can be critical. Only a hospital with a specialist obstetric unit can provide all the emergency facilities that might be needed. Of course, such crises are quite rare. Nevertheless, at the stage when the condition becomes severe—signalled by the onset of proteinuria —it is not possible to predict who will and who will not become dangerously ill. That's why you need to be in hospital until your baby can be safely delivered (see p. 101).

What is toxaemia? Is it a form of blood poisoning?

Toxaemia is an outdated synonym for pre-eclampsia. It implies, quite wrongly, that something toxic has been eaten or that there is a dangerous infection in the bloodstream. Doctors still talk about 'pre-eclamptic toxaemia', largely because it can be shortened to the convenient acronym PET. However, no-one now believes that the disease is caused by toxins (see p. 15).

QUESTIONS ABOUT THE BABY

Why must my baby be delivered early?

As pre-eclampsia is an illness caused by the presence of a sick placenta within the mother's body, it can be cured only by delivery;
and, as the disease is progressive, it always gets worse until delivery
has taken place. When deciding on the timing of delivery, doctors
have to balance the interests of the mother with those of her unborn
baby. If both mother and baby are being adversely affected by the
illness, and the baby is mature enough to survive outside the womb,
those interests coincide. But the balancing act is at its most delicate
when severe illness arises at the very beginning of the third trimester
—or even earlier—when delivery might threaten the baby's survival. Such decisions can be agonizing for all concerned but, as you
might expect, the mother's interests always come first (see p. 103).

Will my baby be normal?

Pre-eclampsia carries no increased risk of malformation. The form
of a baby is determined largely during the first 3 months of pregnancy, which is many weeks before the maternal illness of pre-
eclampsia can possibly set in. The problems for the baby come in the
second half of pregnancy when the placenta begins to fail. But by this
time the baby is fully formed and has only to grow and mature.

There are some very rare fetal chromosomal disorders, causing
severe malformation, which seem to carry an increased risk of pre-
eclampsia. It is also theoretically possible to have two unrelated
problems simultaneously: a pre-eclamptic pregnancy and a malformed baby.

Will my baby suffer brain damage?

This is possible but extremely unlikely. Because the placental blood
flow is reduced in pre-eclampsia, the baby can become short of
oxygen and this can increase the risk of brain damage before, during
or after delivery. It is to guard against such dangers that babies
affected by pre-eclampsia are monitored so closely and so regularly.
If all the observations are normal, it is highly unlikely that a baby
is at risk of brain damage (see p. 104).

**Scans have shown that my baby is 'small for dates':
why is this?**

The most likely reason is that the placenta is not receiving enough
blood from your circulation to supply the baby with all the nutrients
it needs for normal growth. Not all women with pre-eclampsia have
small babies, but the earlier the disease develops the more likely
the baby is to be affected (see p. 82).

Can I help my baby grow by eating more?

No: your diet is not to blame for your baby's restricted growth
because this is essentially a circulatory problem, not a nutritional
one. The nutritional ingredients your baby needs are readily available in your bloodstream but are not reaching the placenta in the
correct concentrations because your uterine blood vessels are too
small, or blocked, or both (see p. 84).

QUESTIONS ABOUT BLOOD PRESSURE

**What do the figures in a blood pressure reading mean, and
which is most important?**

The pressure of blood within your arteries rises and falls with each
heartbeat. The pressure is highest (systolic pressure) while the heart
is contracting, and lowest (diastolic pressure) when it relaxes
between beats. The two figures given in a reading represent the
systolic and the diastolic pressure in the brachial artery supplying
your forearm, as measured on a mercury pressure gauge. Doctors
tend to ascribe more importance to the diastolic reading, but the
systolic pressure may be just as important in pre-eclampsia, and a
reading of 160/80 (high systolic only) should be as much a matter
for concern as one of 135/95 (high diastolic only) (see pp. 33 and
96).

What raises the blood pressure in pre-eclampsia?

The best explanation is spasm in the small arteries. To maintain
blood flow through these constricted vessels, the heart has to pump
blood out at a higher-than-normal pressure (see p. 60).

What is 'pregnancy-induced hypertension'?

In some cases rising blood pressure towards the end of pregnancy signals the onset of pre-eclampsia, but in others it reveals an underlying tendency to chronic hypertension. The term 'pregnancy-induced hypertension' (PIH) is intended to apply to both circumstances and to separate high blood pressure occurring on its own from proteinuric pre-eclampsia. However, many doctors use the terms PIH and pre-eclampsia interchangeably, which is a good reason for abandoning the term (see p. 4).

How can my blood pressure be high when I feel so well?

As a rule, high blood pressure causes no symptoms whatsoever until it reaches a high enough level—usually at or above 200/130 mmHg —for the arteries to be in danger of bursting. This is an extremely rare situation in pregnancy, so how you feel has very little, if any, bearing on the level of your blood pressure (see pp. 64 and 113).

Why does my blood pressure remain high when I have rested and am completely relaxed?

It is a common misconception that you can bring down high blood pressure with rest and relaxation. Blood pressure is controlled by complex mechanisms, most of which are beyond our conscious control. It is true that stresses like anxiety, pain, and lack of sleep can lead to higher pressures, but their absence doesn't guarantee low pressures. This is particularly true with pre-eclampsia, when very powerful forces originating from the sick placenta are combining to drive the blood pressure up. Your blood pressure can be controlled —temporarily—by drugs, but only delivery can restore it to normal (see p. 62).

Can my high blood pressure damage the baby?

No: your baby is not exposed to your blood pressure because it has a totally separate circulatory system. However, your blood pressure is raised because of circulatory problems in the placenta and these problems certainly *can* affect the baby by keeping it short of oxygen and nutrients (see p. 82).

What damage can high blood pressure do to me?

The major risk is that very high pressure could lead to a stroke caused by the bursting of an artery in the brain. For most women the pressure would have to be extraordinarily high—200/130 mmHg or more for several hours—to represent a serious risk, although a small minority have weak spots in their cerebral arteries and are therefore at risk from less extreme pressures.

In pregnancy doctors are concerned about even moderately raised pressures—around the 140/90 level—not because these pressures are dangerous in themselves but because they are often the first sign of pre-eclampsia and an indication for more frequent monitoring (see p. 65).

Why did I suffer eclampsia even though my blood pressure was never very high?

High blood pressure does not cause pre-eclampsia or eclampsia: it is simply one of several effects of the condition. In general the higher the blood pressure the worse the illness; but in a minority of cases serious complications, such as eclampsia, can arise when the blood pressure is only moderately raised—or even normal (see p. 61).

My blood pressure is always higher in hospital than when my community midwife takes it. Wouldn't I be better off at home?

No: the aim of treating pre-eclampsia is not to achieve the lowest possible blood pressure, any more than the aim of treating a serious infection is to get rid of the fever. High blood pressure does not *cause* the problems of pre-eclampsia, so getting it down does not resolve them. It may be true that your blood pressure is higher than it would be at home, but hospital is still the best place for anyone with severe pre-eclampsia (see p. 101).

Would it help if I learned to measure my own blood pressure at home?

It might—providing you have no other signs of pre-eclampsia. Some women suffer from 'labile hypertension', meaning that their blood pressure readings tend to be raised in certain situations, particularly clinics. For such women it can be helpful to demonstrate that pressures taken at home are consistently normal. However, once proteinuric pre-eclampsia has been diagnosed, home monitoring is not such a good idea. For reasons see p. 102.

QUESTIONS ABOUT MEDICATION

Are the drugs used to control blood pressure in pregnancy safe for my baby?

Most drugs can cross the placenta and enter the baby's bloodstream, and so should be prescribed only when absolutely necessary. However, most antihypertensive drugs are tolerated well by unborn babies. Beta-blockers should not be used all the way through pregnancy because they tend to slow fetal growth rates; but this seems not to be a problem in the last month or two. The class of drugs known as ACE inhibitors, are definitely *not* safe towards the end of pregnancy, when they can cause serious, even lethal problems for the baby, such as irreversible kidney failure (see p. 109).

Is it safe to conceive while taking drugs for chronic hypertension?

There is no evidence that any of the drugs currently used to treat chronic hypertension cause fetal malformations. But it is possible that they might cause subtle problems that have yet to be discovered. For this reason your treatment should be continued in the pre-conception period and in early pregnancy only if it is absolutely necessary. By 12 weeks your blood pressure is almost bound to have come down anyway, as pregnancy has naturally antihypertensive effects (see p. 34).

QUESTIONS ABOUT PROTEINURIA

Can the protein in my urine damage the baby?

No: it is a sign of severe pre-eclampsia and therefore of severe placental disease. The problems in the placenta can threaten the baby, but not the proteinuria itself.

What does the symbol NAD mean after a urine test?

This is an acronym for 'nothing abnormal detected'—which means your sample is clear as far as the dipstick test can ascertain.

What does it mean to have one or more 'plusses' of protein in the urine?

One or more 'plusses' recorded after a dipstick urine test means that you have an abnormally high concentration of protein in your urine. This is sometimes a sign of a urinary tract infection but is more often an indication of severe pre-eclampsia, particularly if it occurs in late pregnancy and is preceded by a rise in blood pressure. The more 'plusses' you have—the maximum is four—the greater the concentration of protein in your urine and the more serious your condition is likely to be. However, because these tests measure the *concentration* of protein in your urine, and not the total *amount*, the results tend to vary according to the volume of water in your urine. So if you have two 'plusses' one day and one the next, it does not mean your condition is improving. Once you have been admitted to hospital the dipstick tests are likely to be double-checked by 24-hour urine collections, which measure the total amount of protein in your urine (see pp. 69 and 126).

What does it mean to have a 'trace' of protein in the urine?

Sometimes it means that small amounts of protein are beginning to appear in the urine, giving an early warning of severe pre-eclampsia. But more often it means nothing at all. The dipstick test is prone to false readings and traces of protein are so common and so unlikely to be significant that they should probably be regarded as negative results.

Would it help if I tested my own urine every day at home?

Home urine testing might be reassuring to you—and your doctor —if you have raised blood pressure alone. But once proteinuria has set in, you need to be monitored in hospital (see pp. 101 and 126).

Does my diet affect the protein in my urine?

No: the appearance of protein in the urine usually indicates that the kidneys are becoming 'leaky' and allowing blood proteins, which are normally retained in the body, to escape with the waste products in the urine (see p. 70).

QUESTIONS ABOUT SYMPTOMS

Why did I feel so well when I was actually seriously ill?

Feeling really ill is normally a very late event in pre-eclampsia: it is a sign that the systems of your body have begun to break down and you are at risk of serious complications. If you are still feeling well with severe pre-eclampsia then you are not yet 'ill' in the accepted sense; rather you are standing on the edge of a precipice —in extreme danger but intact. Once you feel really ill you have fallen over the precipice into the abyss. The whole point of being in hospital is to enable doctors to keep you from the abyss (see p. 101).

What caused my terrible headache?

Headache can, although rarely, be a symptom of very high blood pressure; it can also be a side-effect of antihypertensive drugs. Some pre-eclamptic headaches are very similar to migraine: this is logical because migraines originate from circulatory disturbances in the brain, which are also typical of pre-eclampsia and eclampsia. Oedema of the brain, which is an occasional feature of very severe pre-eclampsia, is also known to cause headache (see p. 75).

I had a severe pain just below my chest. What caused this?

This was probably caused by swelling of the liver—normally a late and serious symptom of the disease. Blood tests at the time can reveal liver damage, which abates after delivery (see p. 74).

QUESTIONS ABOUT PREVENTION

Can rest help to prevent pre-eclampsia?

There is no evidence to justify the widespread belief that it can. It is important for all pregnant women not to overstretch themselves in any way; but there is no reason to believe that putting your feet up or even taking to your bed will keep pre-eclampsia at bay.

Can diet help to prevent pre-eclampsia?

A good well-balanced diet is important for the success of *any* pregnancy, but we cannot recommend a specific diet to prevent pre-eclampsia. In Chapter 6 we examined some of the dietary factors currently thought to influence the risk of pre-eclampsia, but these data are still hypothetical. There is good evidence to suggest that dietary supplements reduce the incidence of pre-eclampsia in women with intrinsically poor diets. However, many women suffer pre-eclampsia on exemplary diets, so there is clearly no simple cause-and-effect relationship (see p. 140).

What can I do to prevent pre-eclampsia in my next pregnancy?

There is no simple formula that is guaranteed to work. The most important contribution you can make to the success of your next pregnancy is to collaborate with a systematic programme of antenatal care, which is geared to anticipating any difficulties before they arise. Because of the complexities of pre-eclampsia, it is vital for you to be looked after by a specialist, not just by your GP and midwife (see p. 123).

Is being overweight a factor? Will it help if I get my weight down before conceiving again?

There is no convincing evidence that obesity predisposes women to pre-eclampsia; neither is there any substance in the old-fashioned idea that weight control can prevent pre-eclampsia. The excessive weight gain, which is often a warning sign of the disease, is caused by fluid retention, which has nothing to do with your diet. Obviously, if you are very overweight, it is a good idea to lose weight anyway, but not while you are pregnant or attempting to conceive.

QUESTIONS ABOUT THE FUTURE

Could pre-eclampsia have damaged my health in any way?

Providing you have not suffered any irreversible damage, such as a stroke, the illness itself appears to have no long-term effects. You might have suffered organ damage—particularly of the liver or kidneys—at the height of the illness, but this is reversible in the great majority of cases. However, for some women pre-eclampsia appears to be triggered or aggravated by an underlying medical problem, such as chronic hypertension or kidney disease. In such cases there may well be long-term health problems, but they are caused by the underlying condition, *not* the pre-eclampsia.

Will I suffer pre-eclampsia in my next pregnancy?

After a normal first pregnancy, your risk of pre-eclampsia in the next pregnancy is very low. After a first pregnancy complicated by severe pre-eclampsia, your risk of a severe recurrence is about 1 in 20. However, this risk rises in the presence of other predisposing factors, such as chronic hypertension, multiple pregnancy or a change of partner. If you *don't* suffer a recurrence of pre-eclampsia in your second pregnancy, your risk is lower for any succeeding pregnancy. However, each recurrence increases the risk for subsequent pregnancies (see p. 123).

Can I get pre-eclampsia in a future pregnancy even though all my pregnancies have been normal so far?

Yes, without a doubt. You are most likely to suffer pre-eclampsia in a second or later pregnancy if you've had it before; but a major study of Aberdeen women, followed through their first and second pregnancies, showed that nearly 1 in 150 women whose blood pressures had been entirely normal in their first pregnancies had severe (proteinuric) pre-eclampsia in their second pregnancies.

Will my daughter have an increased risk of pre-eclampsia when she gets pregnant?

Daughters of women who suffered pre-eclampsia have a greater-than-average risk of succumbing themselves. In a family study of women who suffered eclampsia, their daughters were found to have eight times the average risk of eclampsia and three times the average risk of pre-eclampsia in their own first pregnancies. But even with this increased risk, the odds still favour a normal pregnancy.

In my first pregnancy, when I suffered pre-eclampsia, I was carrying a boy. Will I be safer if I conceive a girl next time?

There have been occasional reports suggesting that pre-eclampsia occurs more commonly among mothers carrying boys; these have never been confirmed.

After pre-eclampsia am I more likely to suffer blood pressure problems later in life?

Pre-eclampsia itself does not predispose you to chronic hypertension in later life. However, an in-built tendency to chronic hypertension increases your susceptibility to pre-eclampsia. So many women who have suffered pre-eclampsia do experience blood pressure problems in later life.

Does my risk of suffering pre-eclampsia rise with age?

Yes: but most older women are protected by having had previous pregnancies. The age-related increase in risk for first-time mothers is small, and is not significant until after age 40.

QUESTIONS ABOUT KNOWLEDGE AND INFORMATION

Why can't doctors cure pre-eclampsia?

They can: delivery of the baby and placenta always guarantees a *complete* cure, although the consequences of rare, irreversible compli-

cations cannot be undone. What you mean is why can't they cure
the disease in such a way as to allow the pregnancy to continue?
There are two reasons: first, pre-eclampsia is what is known as an
'end-stage' disease, which doesn't set in until the placenta has suffered irreversible damage. By this stage only a placental transplant
could be expected to put things right—and that's a science fiction
concept at present. Secondly, it is difficult to devise remedies for a
disease so poorly understood as pre-eclampsia, which is why the
acquisition of more knowledge is the most urgent priority for the
future (see p. 000).

Why isn't more information available about pre-eclampsia?

Partly because it is a complex and poorly understood disease, on
which it is difficult for experts to reach a consensus, and partly
because pregnant women and their advisers are all too willing to
collude in the myth of the 'perfect pregnancy' and avoid facing up
to the real risks. We hope this book will pave the way for a more
open and honest approach to the subject (see p. 147).

Why do doctors appear to know so little about pre-eclampsia?

Because it is a tricky, elusive, mysterious, and unpredictable problem; because severe cases are so rare that most obstetricians see only
a few each year—not enough to make them familiar with all aspects
of the disease; because the medical profession has been slow in
facilitating the development of specialist centres in each region;
because more research is desperately needed; because consumer pressure has been curiously lacking (see Chapters 7 and 8).

Glossary

Accelerations (of the fetal heart rate): a healthy temporary increase in the rate, usually coinciding with fetal movements.

Acidosis: excess lactic acid in the baby's bloodstream, normally indicating distress from lack of oxygen (*see also* lactic acid).

Acute atherosis: a build-up of fatty and other deposits that block the maternal spiral arteries carrying blood to the placenta (*see also* spiral arteries).

Amino acids: the basic 'building blocks' from which proteins are made (*see also* proteins).

Amnion: the innermost maternal membrane surrounding the fetus and amniotic fluid (*see also* amniotic fluid).

Amniotic fluid: the fluid or 'liquor' in which the baby floats inside the uterus (*see also* oligohydramnios, polyhydramnios).

Anticonvulsants: a class of drugs used to prevent or control eclamptic and other fits (*see also* diazepam, magnesium sulphate, phenytoin).

Antihypertensives: a class of drugs used to control high blood pressure (*see also* beta-blocking agent, calcium channel blocking agent, hydralazine, methyldopa).

Antioxidant: a substance that delays or inhibits the process of oxidation (*see also* oxidation).

Anuria: complete cessation of urine production, indicating kidney failure (*see also* oliguria).

Aspirin: common painkiller which, in small doses, inhibits the platelet activity thought to contribute to pre-eclampsia.

Beta-blocking agent: a class of antihypertensive drugs that work by inhibiting certain activities of the sympathetic nervous system. Labetalol and atenolol are commonly used in pregnancy (*see also* sympathetic nervous system).

Biophysical profile: A scoring system for assessing signs of fetal health as shown by ultrasound observations.

Braxton Hicks contractions: regular or irregular painless contractions of the uterus that occur throughout pregnancy.

Caesarean section: delivery of the baby through an incision in the abdomen.

Calcium channel blocking agent: a class of antihypertensive drugs, including nifedipine, which work by relaxing and dilating constricted arteries (*see also* nifedipine).

Cardiac output: the volume of blood pumped out by the heart each minute.

Cardiotocography (CTG): a technique for assessing a baby's health in terms of its heart rate pattern (*see also* accelerations, decelerations, variability).

Central venous pressure (CVP): the pressure in the right side of the heart receiving blood from the veins. This measurement indicates whether or not the heart is getting enough blood to function properly.

Cerebral haemorrhage: a bleed into the brain, causing a 'stroke'.

Chlormethiazole: an anticonvulsant drug used to control eclampsia (*see also* anticonvulsants).

Chorionic villi: the basic units of the placenta, across which nutrients and oxygen pass from the mother's bloodstream to her baby's and waste products travel in the opposite direction.

Chronic hypertension: permanently raised blood pressure, which is usually inherited but can also result from kidney or hormonal disorders (*see also* essential hypertension).

Creatinine: a waste product derived from muscles, which is excreted into the urine but can accumulate in the bloodstream if the kidneys are damaged.

Decelerations (of the fetal heart rate): prolonged slowing of the rate, usually during contractions, indicating shortage of oxygen.

Decidua: the inner lining of the pregnant uterus, so called because it is shed at delivery.

Diastolic pressure: the lowest pressure inside an artery, achieved when the heart relaxes between beats (*see also* systolic pressure).

Diazepam: a drug (also known as Valium), which is used to stop eclamptic convulsions (*see also* anticonvulsants).

Disseminated intravascular coagulation (DIC): a dangerous complication of pre-eclampsia in which blood clotting function is so disturbed that inappropriate clots form throughout the circulation, blocking blood flow to essential organs and posing the risk of uncontrollable haemorrhage.

Diuretic: a class of drugs that stimulate the kidneys to produce more urine, sometimes prescribed when oedema becomes dangerous.

Dominant gene: a gene inherited from one parent that masks the corresponding gene inherited from the other parent.

Doppler ultrasound measurements: a technique used to assess blood flow through arteries and veins. During pregnancy it is most useful to determine the normality of flow in the two arteries in the umbilical cord.

Eclampsia: convulsions occurring as the end-stage of pre-eclampsia.

ELLP syndrome: syndrome characterized by *E*levated *L*iver enzymes and *L*ow *P*latelet levels (*see also* HELLP syndrome).

Endothelial cells: the flattened cells lining the inner surfaces of all blood vessels, which may be damaged in pre-eclampsia (*see also* endothelium).

Endothelium: the inner lining of the heart and blood vessels.

Essential hypertension: a form of chronic hypertension for which no cause can be found other than heredity.

Extracellular matrix: the substance in which the cells of the body are embedded.

Factor X: the name used in this book to refer to the, as yet unidentified, substance (or substances) presumed to be released by the placenta in pre-eclampsia and to cause maternal illness.

Fallopian tubes: the two tubes extending outwards from the uterus to the ovaries, in which fertilization takes place.

Fetal breathing: 'practice' breathing movements of the unborn baby's chest and diaphragm; they are a sign of good health.

Fetus: the unborn child.

Fibrin: the insoluble fibrous blood protein that forms a key part of a blood clot (*see also* thrombosis).

Fish oil: a dietary component containing certain fatty acids that inhibit the platelet activity thought to contribute to pre-eclampsia.

Free radicals: potentially destructive substances thought to be produced by ischaemic organs and possibly by ischaemic placentas, which may help to cause the maternal illness in pre-eclampsia (*see also* lipid per-oxides).

Fulminating pre-eclampsia: pre-eclampsia of particularly rapid onset and development.

Fundus of the uterus: the top end of the womb, opposite its opening.

Gestosis: a rough synonym for pre-eclampsia; more commonly used in the rest of Europe than in the UK.

Glomerulus: a microscopic unit of the kidney that filters waste products out of the bloodstream for excretion as urine and which is often damaged in pre-eclampsia; *plural glomeruli*.

Haemolysis: a dangerous complication of pre-eclampsia in which the red cells of the blood burst and release their contents (*see also* HELLP syndrome).

Heart rate: the number of contractions (beats) per minute.

HELLP syndrome: a rare and dangerous variant of pre-eclampsia, comprising widespread clotting, liver damage, and bursting of the red blood cells.

Hydralazine: a fast-acting antihypertensive drug, which works by dilating constricted blood vessels.

Hyperemesis: excessive vomiting, a complication of early pregnancy.

Hypertension: a blood pressure raised above levels considered to be normal.

Hypotension: a blood pressure below levels considered to be normal.

Hypoxia: shortage of oxygen—a common fetal problem in pre-eclampsia.

Interstitial fluid: fluid filling the spaces between cells.

Intervillous space: the space between the chorionic villi of the placenta (*see also* chorionic villi).

Intrauterine growth retardation (IUGR): slower than normal growth inside the womb—a common fetal problem in pre-eclampsia.

Intubation: the insertion of a tube into the windpipe when a general anaesthetic is given in order to keep the airway open.

Ischaemia: an inadequacy of the blood supply.

Lactic acid: a potentially poisonous product of cells that are short of oxygen (*see also* acidosis).

Lipid peroxides: products of free radical activity, whose blood levels may be raised in pre-eclampsia (*see also* free radicals).

Magnesium sulphate: the standard US treatment for preventing eclamptic convulsions. It is not widely used in the UK.

Mendelian inheritance: a theory of heredity (dealing with the interaction of dominant and recessive characteristics) put forward by Gregor Mendel, after whom it was named (*see also* dominant gene, recessive gene).

Methyldopa: an antihypertensive drug that works by inhibiting activity of the sympathetic nervous system and is commonly used in pregnancy because of its excellent safety record (*see also* sympathetic nervous system).

Nifedipine: a fast-acting antihypertensive drug that dilates the blood vessels, so reducing blood pressure.

Oedema: abnormal accumulation of fluid in the tissues, causing swelling.

Oligohydramnios: too little fluid around the baby, a common problem in severe pre-eclampsia (*see also* amniotic fluid).

Oliguria: reduced urine production, which may indicate impaired kidney function (*see also* anuria).

Oxidation: the chemical reaction of a substance with oxygen. Most food is broken down to release energy by oxidation.

Peripheral resistance: the sum of the resistance to blood flow in all parts of the circulation. Resistance is increased if arteries are constricted. If cardiac work increases to maintain output this in turn forces up the blood pressure.

Phenytoin: an anticonvulsant drug that has recently been introduced as a means of preventing eclamptic fits.

Placebo: a harmless, inert substance used in studies to test the effects of different treatments. Because it looks identical to the active substance being tested, neither patient nor doctor need know whether the patient is taking the placebo or the active treatment.

Placenta: the fetal structure at the end of the umbilical cord that joins the baby to its mother and sustains fetal life by supplying nourishment and oxygen and removing fetal waste products.

Placental abruption: a sudden haemorrhage that occurs in the second half of pregnancy or during labour which forcibly and abruptly separates the placenta from its attachment to the inner aspect of the uterus. It is a rare cause of sudden fetal death.

Placental hydrops: retention of fluid in the placenta.

Placental ischaemia: shortage of blood flowing to the placenta, thought to be one of the central problems of pre-eclampsia.

Placentation: the process by which the placenta establishes itself and organizes its blood supply from the mother in the first half of pregnancy. Placentation is normally deficient in pre-eclampsia (*see also* spiral arteries, trophoblast).

Platelets: specialized blood cells that help with clotting and are thought to be unduly active in pre-eclampsia.

Polycythaemia: increase in the number of red blood cells in the blood.

Polyhydramnios: too much amniotic fluid around the baby—a rare problem in pre-eclampsia (*see also* amniotic fluid).

Pre-eclamptic toxaemia (PET): a synonym for pre-eclampsia.

Pregnancy-induced hypertension (PIH): a term introduced to describe high blood pressure appearing at the end of pregnancy; this may signal either early pre-eclampsia or a tendency to chronic hypertension which will become more pronounced in later life.

Prostacyclin: one of a number of very active chemical messengers produced by the body's cells, called prostaglandins. Prostacyclin causes blood vessels to relax and inhibits the aggregation of platelets. Its production is thought to be deficient in pre-eclampsia (*see also* thromboxane).

Proteins: large molecules, built from amino acids. Proteins are the basic components of every cell of the body and perform many vital functions.

Proteinuria: leakage of blood proteins into the urine—a sign of kidney impairment usually caused in pregnancy by severe pre-eclampsia.

Pulmonary oedema: abnormal fluid in the lungs—a rare but dangerous complication of pre-eclampsia.

Recessive gene: a gene inherited from one parent that can only be expressed if the corresponding gene from the other parent is also recessive (i.e. it is masked by a dominant gene from the other parent) (*see also* dominant gene).

Small-for-dates: a baby that is smaller than expected for the maturity of the pregnancy.

Sphygmomanometer: an instrument for measuring blood pressure indirectly in the brachial artery supplying the forearm.

Spiral arteries: the 150 or so tiny uterine arteries that supply the placenta but which are inadequate to the task in pre-eclampsia (*see also* acute atherosis).

Status eclampticus: the condition of continual eclamptic fits failing to respond to treatment.

Stroke volume: the amount of blood pumped from the heart with each beat.

Sympathetic nervous system: a part of the nervous system that controls many bodily functions, including the diameter of blood vessels, by means of hormonal activity.

Syndrome: a disorder that, like pre-eclampsia, can be recognized only by a characteristic grouping of symptoms and signs, not by a specific diagnostic test.

Systolic pressure: the highest pressure inside an artery, attained while the heart is contracting (*see also* diastolic pressure).

Thrombosis: the formation of a blood clot from aggregated blood proteins and platelets (*see also* fibrin).

Thromboxane: one of a number of very active chemical messengers produced by the body's cells, called prostaglandins. Thromboxane causes blood vessels to constrict and platelets to aggregate. Its production is thought to be increased in pre-eclampsia. (*see also* prostacyclin).

Toxaemia: an obsolete term once used to describe not just pre-eclampsia but many other complications of pregnancy.

Trimester: a 3-month period. Pregnancy is conveniently divided into three trimesters.

Trophoblast: the specialized cells of the placenta that form the interface between mother and baby and are responsible for placentation and the two-way passage of oxygen and nutrients, and waste products.

Ultrasound scan: a technique for visualizing inner structures of the body by analysing the echoes of very high-pitched sound.

Urea: a waste product of protein turnover. It accumulates in the blood if the kidneys are damaged in pre-eclampsia, usually after proteinuria develops.

Uric acid: the waste product of the turnover of genetic material. It accumulates in the blood as an early sign of involvement of the kidneys in pre-eclampsia, usually before proteinuria develops.

Uterus: the womb.

Variability (of the fetal heart rate): second-by-second fluctuations in the heart rate—signs of healthy brain activity.

Zona pellucida: the membrane surrounding the fertilized egg.

Index